Living Beyond the Silence

Sharon R. Wells-Simonson

Published by:
Angel Wings Publications, LLC
P.O. Box 5342
Greensboro, NC 27435
www.angelwingsbridge.com
sharon@angelwingsbridge.com

Library of Congress Cataloging–in–Publication Data: 2019910903
Wells-Simonson, Sharon R, 2019
Living Beyond the Silence/Sharon R. Wells-Simonson
1st ed. p. cm.
ISBN-13: 978-0-9848641-0-2
First Printing, 2019
Printed in the United States of America

ACKNOWLEDGEMENTS

To my daughters and granddaughters: Amber, Shahnta,
Sanai, and Khyla,
I love you all so much; you all are my biggest blessings!

To my husband, Ted Simonson,
Thank you for your love, support, encouragement,
and for bringing happiness into my life!

To my mother, Mary E. Newkirk,
You are so beautiful inside and out.
I will forever be grateful for your encouragement,
support, and unconditional love!

To my sister, Rhonda D. Newkirk,
Thank you for always believing in me,
and for being the best Sissy in the world!

To my family...my endless love!

To every person whose life has been affected by abuse,
It's time to live beyond your silence; you are a warrior.
You are beautiful, and you no longer have to live in shame!

Honorary Mention

A book of this nature would not be possible without the creative assistance and support of those who have helped push me toward fulfillment of my dream. Special thanks are given to each of the following individuals:

Book Cover Design: Creative Ankh Designs

Editors: Lorraine Elzia, Anita Levine

Graphic design for book cover: Creative Ankh Designs

Website designer for Angel Wings Bridge Foundation: Creative Ankh Designs

Transcriber for the personal stories, and true-to-life accounts: Eileen Knoud, Lorraine Elzia

Book Contributors:
Lakeisha Shaw Barnes, MA, LPC
Stephen L. Braveman
Nanette M. Buchanan
Lorraine Elzia
Denise Staples
Dr. Nan Wise
J.L. Whitehead

A very special thank you to Lorraine Elzia of *Aveeda Literary Services*; without her help, this project may not have become a reality. I appreciate your patience, creativity, contribution, support, and for believing in me and my dreams for this project. You are, and always will be, heaven sent. On the most challenging of days, when I didn't think I could do this, you created magic; you have helped me bring to life something that I know will save lives and inspire victims to heal. For that I am truly grateful.

An extended heart-filled show of love and thanks to all those who touched my life and helped me grow, whose names are not mentioned above. Your placement in my life has been a gift from God, and you know your importance; even if I have failed to say it, or mention you by name. Please blame it on my head and not my heart. There is no way I can ever give full recognition to all who have touched my life or helped me make my dreams a reality; but to all the silent soldiers who went to war with me in this battle…to you – my fearless angels along this mission, I say thank you.

BOOK TESTIMONIALS

"In sharing her story, Sharon R. Wells-Simonson beautifully captures the terror that drives victims to silence; but more importantly, she also conveys with wit, fierceness, raw heart, and vulnerability, the journey back to her voice. Even more wonderfully, Sharon binds within these pages the heroes and heroines who refused, like her, to remain silent. Particularly important are the stories of men and people of color who are all too often egregiously passed over.

If we are to put an end to the epidemic that childhood sexual trauma is, we must continue to raise our voices and witness the stories of others; and by way of sharing how we heal, we will foster hope and social change. This book is a potent antidote."

~ Rachel Grant, Sexual Abuse Recovery Coach, Author of Beyond Surviving: The Final Stage in Recovery from Sexual Abuse

******

"Relationships are, and have always been, our human universal language. This truly incredible book is written as a brilliant lighthouse source of wholeness; solvently beckoning and reaching toward the silent, never spoken for, tarnished lives of those who have been broken down by hurtful sexual touches, deceiving deviant persuasions, and worst of all...a 'soul-invasive-attacking-person-influenced virus' which is squelching, capturing, and crippling the inner innocence and goodness of young victims. This is mostly a misunderstood epidemic; and those who actually are willing to thoroughly face the ongoing reality of this horrific scourge, find that it happens within relationships of which, in most all cases, these littlest ones had no choice other than to trust.

Sharon, here and now, explores and magnifies, with genius realization and prophet-like wisdom, the supports of a dawning community; an un-silenced and most effectively (especially here in American society) uncensored and uncovered voices, all gathering like a wondrous choir through the rainbow spectrum of God's children. This book will be *light bright* enough to shine into a hurting and long-suffering sexually abused child's past darkness. Look now to this lighthouse and find your hope-path brightened! Here comes healing; with Dominique, Nan, Sharon, and many others in your own relationships with yourself, with others, and even those who you never imagined healing could be possible."

~Dr. David Cunha, Licensed Addictions Therapist, Doctorate in Pastoral Counseling, Tree of Life Counseling, Greensboro NC

******

"I wholeheartedly recommend *Living Beyond the Silence* by Sharon R. Wells-Simonson. As a fellow survivor of childhood sexual abuse (CSA), and as the NAASCA founder, I found the descriptions of Sharon's experiences hauntingly familiar, even though I am a male. There is hope here in the honest and well-written divulging of Sharon's secrets and the secrets of others. This book educates us of spiritual journey and of recovery. It's often surprising to newcomers when they learn how similar the feelings, thoughts, and decisions of victims can be; even though there are many different ways to be abused and traumatized.

We often keep the damage done to us as secrets. We fear discovery, feel ashamed, accept responsibility (inappropriately), and think no one will ever understand. In adolescence and early adulthood, the results of childhood trauma likewise result in patterns of behaviors – compulsions, addictions, trouble with relationships, and a general sense of unworthiness that we hope won't be noticed by others. We work hard to cover it up. But newcomer survivors will find themselves in the pages of this book, and will no doubt educate those who are uninformed on the many issues of childhood sexual abuse and its trauma."

~ Bill Murray, NAASCA founder and CEO

Table of Contents

FOREWORD

It is with absolute delight that I write the foreword to this edition of Sharon's brave and brilliant book. Sharon's journey has been one of extraordinary healing and transformation. When she first showed up for therapy sixteen or so years ago, she was a young woman struggling with a difficult life. A survivor of sexual abuse, Sharon dealt with significant, and often crushing, depression which she tried, at times, to manage with substances that led only to deeper suffering.

Spiraling deeper in despair about her failed relationships, and the difficult years of dealing with the demands of being a single parent and grandparent while holding down a full-time job, Sharon often self-medicated as a way to ease her pain. The tragedy of her story is that it isn't unlike that of many others who have been sexually abused; but her ability to turn her life around is a victory for others to try and achieve.

In spite of the challenges she was facing, Sharon found a way to address the baggage that was weighing her down mentally and emotionally. With faith, perseverance, and counseling, she found an incredible passion for obtaining healing and wholeness in spite of her pain. In her journey to become whole, Sharon learned to listen and love herself; a lesson that all abuse survivors ultimately need to incorporate into their lives in order to heal. Not only has she overcome her own challenges, but Sharon has created a gentle tsunami wave of healing for her entire family—forgiving those who had harmed her—and sourcing an even larger swell of healing energy for those whose lives she will touch through this book and in her work as an advocate for victims of abuse.

Living Beyond the Silence, tells Sharon's story and the story of others like her. It is an avenue for survivors to know that they are not alone in their pain, their thoughts, and their actions. Often we cannot prevent bad things from happening to us, but we don't have to allow pain and misery to define who we are. Through the voices of others like her, and with resources that bring about internal change, Sharon has put together a tool for healing; one that lets survivors know that they are not alone and that there is hope for their lives.

With help to manage adversity, we can overcome even the most hurtful situations. The key is in recognizing that we are bruised, so that we can find help to fix that which is broken. There is an incredible healing power within the soul; but steps have to be taken in order for the healing to begin. The work that Sharon has done to overcome her abuse serves as an incredible role model for others who hopefully will follow in her footsteps of forging their own paths to recovery. A woman who was once lost and in the pit of despair has now mended relationships, created joy and health, cultivated a loving marriage, and is now on the road to become a professional expert on the topic of overcoming sexual abuse. *Living Beyond the Silence,* is her gift to others who want and need healing. Although I started as Sharon's therapist, I can joyfully say I am now her dear friend and will always be. She has moved past being victimized, and has become a resource in helping others do the same. Sharon is a magnificent fellow traveler.

Dr. Nan Wise, Ph.D.
Licensed Psychotherapist
Certified Sex Therapist, AASECT
Certified Relationship Specialist, The American Psychotherapy Association
Cognitive Neuroscience Researcher, Psychology, Rutgers-Newark
Fellow, The American Psychotherapy Association
Fellow, The National Board for Clinical Hypnotherapists
Board Certified Diplomate, The American Board of Examiners in Social Work

Monsters can only live in the dark; bringing their horrors to light strips them of their tormenting power, making them weak, while giving the victim strength. Sexual abuse is an everyday occurrence perpetrated by individuals from all walks of life. I have chosen to withhold the names and identities of my abusers. This decision is based on my desire to respect the relationships of the people I love and whose lives would be negatively impacted if names were revealed. Finding a way to transform from victim to victor, and reach empowerment beyond abuse is the message; revelation of my perpetrators' identities is irrelevant. The most valuable benefits received along this journey have been learning how to heal, forgive, and love myself; those are the blessings of wisdom that I wish to pass along to others.

~ Sharon R. Wells-Simonson

The Silent Voice in Fear

I feared the darkness, before I knew I was not alone

I feared the sound of the footsteps, before I knew you were coming

Into my room, into my life, into my small world, I feared for my sacred space

I lost my voice, before I understood who I was, who I was to be

I feared the whispers, the tone of the voice, the darkness, whenever I was alone

I feared your whispers, "You are sweet," "You are pretty," "You are mine," "I

love you"

I feared the touch, the hug, the feelings, the confusion

I lost my voice, before I knew, I was special if only to me

I feared what you said was okay, my private place, you pleasured the taste

I feared, I cried, you pleaded, you begged, my voice was my only, my all

I feared, I told, I yelled, I screamed, my silent voice fell on deaf ears

I lost my voice, before I knew, there were more like me

A Silent Voice in Fear

I fear, for those in the dark, alone

I fear, they will grow to hate who they are,

before they understand who they were

I fear, they will be afraid to love, because of THAT touch

I fear their voice will not be heard

I fear they will listen to the whispers, "Be pretty," "Be sweet"

Be his, be hers, but never understand real love

I fear their voice will not be heard

I fear for their private space, the confusion, the personal intrusion

It repeats for me, it repeats for them, it happens for so many more

The Silence has been Broken

I Now Speak for All

Nanette M. Buchanan - © 2019

Introduction

For many victims, healing from child sexual abuse is like peeling back an onion; attempting to discard the hurt, shame, and pain that was inflicted upon them. It is a constant effort to remove layer after layer of tears and heartache in order to mend the bruised and tormented feelings surrounding the core. As a survivor of childhood sexual abuse, it has not been easy for me to move beyond the scars of my abuse. Healing does not happen overnight, but it is possible to move beyond the trauma. It is not uncommon for victims to believe they are responsible for the abuse; especially when it happens to young children. Child sexual abuse strips the victim of their innocence and leaves them feeling like damaged goods. Innocent victims grow up believing that they are damaged and have done something bad and unforgivable.

That's a heavy burden for anyone to carry; which is why I was angry for many years for being robbed of my self-worth and dignity. My dreams of becoming the person I had always dreamed of being were stolen. I spent years avoiding the details of my abuse, and I medicated myself with self-destructive behaviors and failed relationships. My life was interrupted. I didn't believe in myself, and I had no self-esteem, so I didn't raise the bar higher. Instead, I settled into wearing a mask that hid my insecurities while I perfected a false persona. I would look at other people and always felt that everyone else was better than me. I never felt that I measured up to anyone.

In my career, I couldn't seem to find my niche. Although I tried many ventures, each one would end the same. I would start something and then lose interest, and that was the end of that. I had become the "Jack of all Trades" and the master of none. I literally ran in circles chasing my tail. Through my frustration, I would self-medicate, then get clean. I would make progress, and only after a short while, repeat the same sick cycle all over again. Any progress that I made, I sabotaged it and had to begin again. With many failures underneath my belt, something inside me wouldn't allow me to give up. Self-worth was just so hard to grasp, but I believed that if I didn't give up, one day I would love myself.

Personally, I'm not even sure if a person can ever completely heal from sexual abuse. I believe, however, that over time, you get to a better place if you address it and begin working on yourself. For me, and I am sure for many others, the abuse damaged me down to my core. Although I went into therapy in my early twenties, I danced around the details of my abuse. I focused more on the after-effects such as my drug abuse, failed relationships, and depression. It wasn't until I was in my forties that I actually started doing the work necessary concerning the sexual abuse itself.

I was making progress with my therapist, but little did I know that it would take another decade to peel away more layers of the sexual abuse. I continued finding comfort in what was familiar, yet unproductive. Through continued therapy, I started the process of forgiving myself and my abusers. Loving yourself and feeling worthy can take a lifetime, but it surely is possible.

My "A-ha" moment came at fifty-something when I was experiencing anxiety from playing catch up with my life. Because I suffered for so many years, I felt like I was running out of time in my career, and in my personal life. Although my marriage was wonderful, and relationships with my family had been repaired, I still felt like there was so much more that I needed to do. There were times when I felt purposeless, especially while at work. Deep inside, I knew I had so much more to offer, but my career was going nowhere. Each position was just another dead-end job. Although I was grateful and blessed to have a job, I've always known that I was smart and capable of doing greater things. However, I take full responsibility for keeping myself stagnated for so many years. I wasn't blind to the fact that the sexual abuse was the reason for my ill-fated, repetitious life.

Now in my fifties, I have started to live; no more self-medicating or running from my past. I embrace my journey, although it is not the one I had imagined. I have been broken, and today I am still putting pieces together. Most days I believe in myself and I will continue the journey of becoming whole. Although there are days when the remnants of my abuse seep into my mind, I have learned to utilize positive self-talk, dust myself off, and keep it moving. Forgiving is truly possible, but the memories of the abuse will never be forgotten.

But what I cannot wrap my head around is, *what makes a person think it's alright to violate another person solely for their own sexual pleasure? What is the fascination of stealing something as precious as someone's spirit, dignity, and self-respect? What is so captivating about desecrating another human being, that it causes someone to destroy their own legacy, family, and their own life? What's the reward in exhibiting that kind of destructive behavior? Is the allure of individual sexual gratification really that strong? And if so, when will we, as a society, truly recognize the magnitude of the problem and the lasting effect it has on victims?*

In 2011, when I first released *Without Permission, A Spiritual Journey to Healing*, sexual abuse was still an issue no one wanted to discuss. Those who did talk about it, often did so with a sense of shame, as if they had done something wrong. Sadly, society has programed us to blame the victim instead of placing the guilt where it belongs – upon the perpetrator. For centuries, society has always turned a blind eye and a deaf ear to this type of abuse. Because of its shameful nature, countless numbers of families with incidences of abuse have chosen to sweep those occurrences under the rug. Typically, people find it too uncomfortable and too painful to talk about. Sexual abuse is treated as a taboo subject, when in actuality, it's so much more than that…it's a crime, and it's time that our society give it the label that it deserves.

Just in recent years, victims have begun breaking their silence, creating movements, and demanding that society open its eyes to what was often deemed the skeleton in the closet for most families.

Statistically, some victims try to self-medicate the pain of sexual abuse by seeking comfort in drugs, alcohol, and promiscuous behavior in order to numb their suffering. Unfortunately, in most cases, drugs and alcohol will only make matters worse; leading to a self-destructive lifestyle and possibly fatal consequences. Mental health issues have been linked as effects of sexual abuse in some victims.

The effect of sexual abuse not only affects the victims, but it also negatively impacts the lives of their families as well. Due to the trickledown effect of sexual assault – from perpetrator to victim, from victim to their loved ones, from those loved ones down to everyone they come in contact with – we can no longer ignore or keep silent about this issue that is plaguing our communities. Ultimately, through education, further research and proper treatment, we can diminish the ripple effect that stems from the immoral action of one person, but affects so many. Childhood sexual abuse is a traumatic experience that has many consequences throughout the person's life.

Often when we have conversations about sexual abuse in any form, people will admit that they know someone who has been abused. That's a sad reality, and the list of names could go on and on. But the real question is, why?

Why is sexual abuse so ramped? Why aren't more people outraged? Why didn't the perpetrator know that when they took something that didn't belong to them, that it would cause their victim a lifetime of pain and sorrow? Did they know that their uninvited touch would redirect another person's life to somewhere they didn't choose to go? Did they even care? Do we?

I think we do. I think we are making strides to fix the problem and it starts with first admitting that the problem exists; and having done that, we next need to address why.

In the pages that follow are true stories of male and female victims, and how child sexual abuse has negatively impacted their lives. Children of every gender, age, race, ethnicity, background, socioeconomic status and family structure are at risk. No child is immune. The stories never get old and will always be a reminder of how much work still needs to be done to protect our children. I have also chosen to re-tell a portion of my life story from victim to survivor.

When I released my first book, that project helped me to begin my healing journey. It was a vulnerable time in my life, but it was important that my voice be heard. I was not just speaking for myself, but for others who were unable to break their silence. Now that I have removed the cloths of shame and guilt, I speak from a place of strength and perseverance. I will never forget my past, but I've started new chapters in my life; ones that are filled with peace, self-love, and dignity.

Unfortunately, even when victims do find the courage to break their silence, the hurt and pain still exist, leaving a gaping hole in their lives. My hope is that *"Living Beyond the Silence"* will be a guide to help victims reclaim their lives and begin their journey to healing. Because sexual abuse is so complicated, there isn't a quick fix that will erase all of the hurt and pain. Ultimately, my hope is that the information and resources provided in this book will help you better understand the effects of abuse, and help you free yourself from self-imprisonment.

What is Sexual Abuse?
THE MORRIS CENTER, Revised 7/99, www.ascasupport.org

Sexual Abuse is defined as any sexual act directed at a child involving sexual contact, assault, or exploitation. Sexual abuse is divided into two categories: contact and non-contact. Acts of contact child sexual abuse include fondling, rape, incest, sodomy, lewd or lascivious acts, oral copulation, intercourse, and penetration of a genital or anal opening by a foreign object. Examples of non-contact sexual abuse include exhibitionism, presentation of pornographic pictures, telling of sexual stories, allowing the child to witness adult sexual relations, treating the child in a sexually provocative way, or promoting prostitution in minors.

Physical signs that may suggest sexual abuse of children include sexually transmitted diseases; genital discharge or infection; physical injury, irritation of the oral, anal or genital areas; pain when urinating or defecating; difficulty walking or sitting due to genital or anal pain; and stomachaches, headaches, or other psychosomatic symptoms. Again, most, if not all, of these symptoms can result from other, non-abuse related causes or conditions. Please keep this in mind as you evaluate your own history. Behavioral signs that may result from sexual abuse include age inappropriate sexual behavior with peers or toys; excessive curiosity about sexual matters; overly advanced understanding of sexual behavior (especially in younger children); compulsive masturbation, prostitution or promiscuity; and incontinence (in the case of anal intercourse). Once again, these symptoms may be the result of other occurrences, and you should be wary of jumping to any conclusions. Concern about, and awareness of, sexual abuse has grown dramatically in recent years as numerous public surveys have reported its pervasiveness. It is currently estimated that up to one third of all women, and up to one seventh of all men over the age of twenty-one, have been sexually abused as children.

Sexual abuse may be the final skeleton in the family closet; one that has been obscured for years, or even generations behind a veil of secrecy and denial. Thanks to the emergence of the adult survivor movement, men and women who have suffered from childhood sexual abuse for years as children are now breaking their silence about their secret. Sometimes abused children think that if they couldn't stop the abuse, then they were at least partially responsible for it. Trends in state laws challenge this kind of thinking. For example, in California, if the child victim is under the age of fourteen, any sexual contact with an adult is presumed to be sexual abuse, even if the child has purportedly consented. In the case of child victims over the age of fourteen who may have consented to the sexual contact, the issue is determined by looking (*Survivor to Thriver*, Page 39 ©1995 THE MORRIS CENTER, Revised 7/99, ascasupport.org) at a number of factors, including the age of the adult, the nature of the relationship, and the emotional maturity of the child. Some teenagers under the age of eighteen may not have sufficient psychological maturity to consent to a relationship with someone much older, while others may be deemed to have consented. The determination will vary in each situation.

There are many factors that place children at risk for sexual abuse, especially in an era of high divorce rates and blended families. Children are most likely to be sexually abused between the ages of 8-12. Girls are more at risk for sexual abuse than boys (statistics show one out of every three girls compared to one out of every seven boys). Girls who are abused are more likely to live in a blended family or with a single mother who is employed outside the home. When a natural father is the abuser, the girl's mother is often absent or uninvolved for some reason. She may be disabled, ill, working outside of the home, or alcoholic. Factors such as these may result in less than adequate care-giving and a lack of parental authority. The parents' marital relationship may be in discord, and the parents may be avoiding dealing with each other. Ever so gradually, the father may begin to place the girl in the role of his wife.

Sexual abuse also happens to boys, although not to the extent reported for girls. Boys are more likely to be abused by adult males, teenage siblings, and other older boys known to the victim. Some male victims might later point to this sexual abuse as the cause of confusion about their sexual identity. When the molester is female, boys are confused about how to interpret the experience. Is it sexual abuse or sexual opportunity? Because boys are socialized to want sex, cultural norms often cloud their perceptions of the experience. Because boys are supposed to be "tough" and able to defend themselves, they may be disinclined to speak up about having been taken advantage of. In many cases, it may be a more convenient psychologically for them to interpret their abuse as a "conquest" rather than a victimization. But the conflicts do not go away just because the abuse is cast in a positive light.

Incest between mother and son is every bit as harmful as father-daughter incest. Mother-son incest is usually the outgrowth of a long-established seductive relationship that may then evolve into overt sexual relations when the boy reaches puberty and begins experiencing his own sexual awakening. This is an important dynamic that touches on issues of emotional abuse as well.

Although some children may feel responsible, the responsibility always rests with the parent to set appropriate standards of behavior. In cases of mother-son incest, the mother is almost always incapacitated as a parent due to addictions, severe emotional problems, or her own unresolved childhood sexual abuse (*Survivor to Thriver*, Page 40 ©1995 THE MORRIS CENTER, Revised 7/99, www.ascasupport.org).

There are many factors that can influence the degree of impact of sexual abuse on a child. A child who has been abused by more than one offender is likely to be more traumatized because the repetition of the abuse reinforces the child's attitude that she/he is somehow responsible. The type of sexual contact can also be significant. Intercourse can have more serious consequences than fondling or exposure to pornography. When aggression or violence is used to force sex, the impact is even more negative because the child feels fear and greater loss of control, as compared to more seductive molestation in which persuasion and manipulation are employed. When children participate to some degree in the sexual contact or are unable (as is usually the case) to find a way to prevent the abuse from happening, the guilt and shame over their involvement often causes severe consequences. If there were some pleasurable sensations from the contact (common when the abuse involves fondling), children often interpret their feelings as evidence of their culpability and responsibility. Children do not usually understand that the responsibility for preventing sexual expression of affection lies with the parent or adult.

In cases where the sexual abuse occurs outside of the home, the reaction of the family is paramount in shaping the degree of impact on the child. When the family is supportive, gets immediate help for the child, and avoids any blaming or stigmatization, the long-term effects can be lessened. However, when the family does not understand, blames the child for the sexual abuse, or is unable to accept that the child was victimized, the impact can be truly devastating because the family's reaction confirms the child's worst fears: that she/he did something wrong, or did not do enough to prevent the sexual abuse. In these cases, the family members become co-conspirators in the abuse because, in failing to give the child what she/he needs during a time of tragedy, they may do far more damage to the child than the abuser did. It is no surprise that children will feel stigmatized by the sexual abuse if their families treat them with disdain and disgust. Sexual abuse outside the family may have actually increased during the last twenty years because more children are being cared for in daycare centers, afterschool programs, and juvenile institutions.

There has been a rash of stories of sexual molestation in daycare centers across the country, although proving guilt in these cases has often been unsuccessful. There are even three "pro-pedophilia" organizations operating in North America, all dedicated to finding and maintaining sexual relationships with young girls and boys. With the explosion of the adult film industry, there is evidence that child pornography rings are proliferating. It is estimated that upwards of half a million (*Survivor to Thriver*, Page 41 ©1995 THE MORRIS CENTER, Revised 7/99, www.ascasupport.org) children are involved in these activities. Teenage runaways, many of whom end up on the streets hustling for food and money, are likely targets for sexual abuse and exploitation. Unfortunately, the effects of child sexual abuse will not be fully felt until today's child victims grow up to become tomorrow's adult survivors.

Part I
Sharon's Story

Chapter One
Secrets of Summer Bring the Birth of a Warrior

In retrospect, I realize that our childhood years are the most impressionable and critical years in our lives. Every experience we have has a way of molding us into the person we become later in life. Good or bad, healthy or dysfunctional, those experiences become the potter and we are merely the clay. Moving away from my family in Philadelphia to a new home in New Jersey at the age of four years old when my parents married was very devastating to me. New Jersey was an unfamiliar place where I had no family or friends. While in elementary school, I was constantly being bullied by my classmates because of my skin color being so different from theirs, being well dressed, and what we called back then, having "good hair."

My parents knew how much I loved spending time with my family in Philly, and a way to keep me out of fights during the summer months, they would send me to my grandparents' house. As I grew up, I learned that life has a way of tainting even the most beautiful memories. Amongst all the love I was receiving from being around my family, that same family environment opened up a path that eventually led to my abuse. My guard was down due to the fact that abusers sometimes wear the robe of trust. Abusers sometimes hide behind the mask of family or friends.

It was during two different summer breaks that I was sexually molested by two different men. I was almost eight the first time it happened, and I was barely aware of my changing body. Apparently, others were noticing changes in my body and taking notes for their own pleasure.

I was alone, that first time, with someone I trusted. I didn't think about it too much when he suggested I go with him into the kitchen. I had no reason to be leery of being alone with him; after all, he was a family friend. Once inside the kitchen, I watched, in shock, as he leaned against the refrigerator and greased his genitals with *Royal Crown* petroleum jelly. I knew that men and boys had different genitals than I had, but I had never seen a penis before in my life. *Royal Crown* changed all that for me. As he stroked himself using the refrigerator as leverage to hold his body up, I noticed his penis beginning to grow. All I could do was stare, not knowing what to do. I wasn't sure what was going on as he smiled a wicked grin in my direction, continuing his up and down strokes while applying the jelly on himself. I looked around the kitchen wondering, what, if anything, his actions had to do with me.

Everything became clearer when he positioned me directly in front of him, pulled my panties down to my ankles, and slid himself back and forth between my legs. He made grunting sounds, which got faster and louder as he continued to slide back and forth. After a few minutes, I felt a sticky substance drip down my legs, and then he withdrew from between my legs. It was over.

He said very little to me as he pulled up his pants and reached into his pants pockets. I remember that he was too tall for me to look him eye-to-eye in the face. I do remember that after he was done and had pulled up his pants, he cleaned off the substance from my legs with a kitchen towel, pulled up my panties, and gave me some change out of his pocket to go to the candy store.

The fact that he never told me not to tell anyone about what happened was a given; the money he gave me was payment for my silence. I accepted it shamefully, sure that I must have done something wrong even if I wasn't sure what it was. I tried to make sense of it all as I ran to the corner store. I allowed the blackmailing treats of my molester to silence me.

I knew that what happened was dirty somehow, but I was too young to understand that I had just been molested. I couldn't make the connection in my head. All I knew was that my otherwise care-free summer had just been compromised along with my innocence. I didn't know exactly what secret I was being paid to keep, but what-ever it was, I was sure it was shameful. It felt nasty, and it made me feel unclean. That was enough for me to know that what happened was not right.

I didn't know the names for male and female genitals, but I knew they were always referred to as private parts. That meant they were private, not to be shown or touched by anyone. My abuser had shown me his private part before he had seen or touched mine. My gut told me that his doing so wasn't right, which confused me. I had trusted him.

Why had he done this?
Was it my fault?
Did I somehow make him think it was okay to treat me the way he did?

I went back home to New Jersey at the end of that summer a changed girl with a different perspective on trust. At the age of eight, my view of the world had been tainted. I never told a soul about what happened that day. I saw my abuser a few times during the year when my parents took me to Philadelphia for family visits, but I always acted as if nothing happened. I never said a word. Even now, many years later, *Royal Crown* petroleum jelly brings back memories I have tried so hard to forget. If I succeeded in denying what happened by burying it in the back of my mind, the sight or smell of *Royal Crown* is still a little trigger which is always enough to bring it all flooding back to the forefront of my mind.

I was molested again during another summer break about a year later, when I was almost nine. My second abuser was also someone I knew and trusted. I went to his house to visit his sister, but quickly found out he was the only one home at the time. Trusting him because I had known him and his family for a very long time, when he invited me in to his bedroom, I went without apprehension.

Once in his room, I sat on the bed and we talked for a little bit about nothing in general other than small talk. I was completely surprised when he laid me back on the bed and got on top of me. He transformed from a position of being the brother of my friend, to being a sexual partner. He rubbed his hands all over my body and kissed me as if I were a willing partner. Feeling shocked and very, very dirty and ashamed at what he was doing to my body, I quickly managed to free myself and get out of the house. I pushed him off of me and ran until my legs and my lungs could no longer deal with the extra exertion on both. I finally made it to a place where I could sit and gather both my breath and my thoughts.

I never told anyone about what he had done. For many years, I also succeeded in blocking the memory of it out of my mind. I didn't put a label on it when it happened. I was too young to give the experience a definition; but in looking back, I realize now that what he did was molest me that day. Although he never penetrated me, he violated me in a way I'll never forget. A way that I didn't consent to, and one that changed the way I viewed myself. I'm sure, too, that he knew exactly what he was doing at the time he did it. My feelings meant nothing to him. They rarely do when it comes to predators and prey. He got what he wanted, which was to do exactly what he did, as he took advantage of me in the worst possible way.

After that incident, my body began to develop. I was going through the puberty stage. My breasts were in a weird stage and had begun protruding, which embarrassed me more than I can ever say. They were so noticeable that the boys began calling me, *Torpedo*. I started putting Band-Aids over my nipples in an attempt to avoid the unwanted attention.

At the age of twelve, somehow history has a way of repeating itself. Little did I know that what happened to me during those summers in Philly was about to happen again. My abuser, John, whose identity I've chosen not to disclose, was a family friend who molested me whenever the opportunity presented itself. I did my best to avoid him in every way possible. Unfortunately, he was so connected to my family and me that it was impossible for me not to have interaction with him. It started out by what I thought was an innocent kiss of just touching lips until he tried sliding his tongue into my mouth.

After the initial sliding of the tongue, he always seemed to want to give me a kiss when he greeted me. He was someone that my family and I knew and loved very much. I shunned it off and made myself believe that I was imagining what was happening, and that molestation was not the case concerning him and me. Then one day, while I was alone with him, he kissed me again. At that time, not only did he slide his tongue in to my mouth, but he fondled my breast too. As his fingers fumbled with my budding breasts, his actions brought back repulsive feelings of those summers spent in Philadelphia. I did not want to believe that the same thing was happening to me all over again. Somewhere in the back of my mind, I knew that things were just the same, only in a different, more grown-up body. I could not respond to his advances, even though I knew what he was doing was wrong. When he touched my body, I froze in the same fear I had before. I wanted to scream, but no sounds would come out of my mouth. I was traumatized by what he was doing to me. He had severed the bond between us. I couldn't imagine what he could be thinking that would allow him to be so selfish in his actions. I felt ashamed, and thought that if I told anyone about it, they would not believe me, so why take the chance on causing myself more shame.

There I was once again, having to bury yet another secret and bear more shame. I continued to blame myself. I felt like I must be doing something which caused men to act in a manner that everyone, even someone of my age, knew to be wrong. No one in the family had a clue that John was touching my body in places and ways he had no permission to do.

John even went so far as to check my private parts to see if I was still a virgin. It was important in his mind that I was. I tried convincing him that my virginity was in tack, but he made it a point of fondling me anyway to inspect for himself. He wanted to make sure I was still pure. Each time John touched me, I sank further and deeper into a black hole. I could never understand why God was allowing me to be a victim in that way. By the time I turned fourteen, concealing the secret of my continuous molestation was tearing me apart inside.

While enduring the molestation, I still had the ongoing problem of being bullied at school. I didn't know how to find comfort from the bullying, and I was tired of running home each day. I felt it was time for me to start standing up for myself. There was a feeling stirring inside of me as if there was someone inside me who was screaming to get out. That person, who I did not know existed, showed up one day during my gym class in seventh grade. I had gotten into an altercation with one of my classmates over something minor. Before I knew it, we were scuffling outside on the track field. My rage, which had built up over several years, was the product of repressed mental and physical abuse. It found a way to unleash itself. The person inside of me who had been locked away found a way to emerge from the depth of her hiding place. I blacked out during the fight; all that I could remember afterwards was the two teachers who pulled me off of my classmate. When I saw that she had a bloody nose, I knew that I was in big trouble.

At that point, I felt bad about my classmate's nose, but it felt good to finally stand up for myself. The new, unfamiliar person from deep inside me was bold, sassy, and courageous; the total opposite of me. I welcomed her emergence. It was liberating. It didn't take long before I allowed her presence to take over and let the timid and fearful person that I was, fade into the background. We were one person, but I allowed her to take the forefront and protect us both.

I vowed to no longer be afraid; my perception about the world was that it was a battlefield. I was on guard, and ready to attack anyone who I thought was out to hurt me. In my mind, most people were the enemy and I was ready for war. I kept a serious look on my face and rarely cracked a smile; which quickly became my defense mechanism. I wanted to numb my pain. I was unhappy, and I just didn't want to feel anything anymore. I remained that way from that moment on through high school.

In middle school, I started experimenting with serious drugs. Attending *get high* parties was where I found a variety of drugs. Someone from school would have a party at their house while their parents were at work. We would all cut school to go and hope that their parents wouldn't come home early. It was at those parties where I was first introduced to drugs like THC, Hash, Acid, Cocaine, as well as many others. Cocaine always seemed to be my drug of choice.

My parents noticed the change in me, and saw that my unpredictable behavior was spiraling out of control. It wasn't long before they grew overly concerned because I was not communicating with them at all. They became frustrated, and made an appointment for me to see a psychiatrist, hoping to get some answers to my behavior. They knew I was acting differently, but they had no clue I was using drugs. What they were also clueless about was that I was angry with them too because they had not figured out, on their own, what was troubling me. I refused to open up to the doctor, which my parents eventually realized was a waste of time in trying to pursue. They were not getting any closer to figuring out my problems, nor was the doctor. After a few more sessions and still no progress being made, my parents canceled the rest of the appointments and we never went back again.

The pressure of trying to figure out who I was, and what I wanted to do with my life, was overwhelming. I based my identity on who everyone else thought I should be. At that time, the only thing that mattered to me was staying numb in order to keep the secrets that were still tormenting me buried as far down inside as possible.

Most of the time, I felt like I wore an invisible sign on my forehead that said, "Damaged Goods." I was convinced that the world could see that I was tainted. There were so many times when I wanted to tell someone what was happening, or just scream it out so loud that some-one, anyone, would make him stop. However, my hidden shame pre-vented me from doing that. It kept me in a place where I had no idea how to make him stop or how to free myself from his reign.

The pain from the abuse, and from concealing it, was so unbear-able that my mind often felt like a pressure cooker ready to explode. I felt alone and abandoned; like there was no one to protect me, least of all myself. I experienced a lot of headaches during that time be-cause the burden of my mental distress was overwhelming.

That year, I became enraged and unwilling to continue protecting the man who apparently felt entitled to violate my body whenever he wanted. One evening, I started praying. I asked God to give me the courage and strength to tell my mother what was happening to me. I knew I could put my trust in her and I hoped she would believe me. A few hours later, my prayers were answered. God gave me the strength I needed to make my decision. He told me everything would be okay. He assured me that it was time to stop hiding the source of my pain.

Armed with the comfort from above, nothing and no one could stop me from revealing the secret that was causing me so much shame. That night, I waited until everyone was asleep before I tiptoed into my parents' bedroom. I gently tapped my mother's shoulder to wake her as she lay asleep in bed. I told her I needed to talk to her about something really important.

Her eyes piqued with curiosity as she slowly rose from her bed. It wasn't an every-day occurrence for her daughter to say she had something important to talk about, and I could feel her motherly concern. Still groggy from being awakened from her sleep, she followed me downstairs. I made sure that I turned the light to the dim setting to hide my face before sharing the most shameful secret of my life.

We sat a few inches from each other on the couch. She was just about to ask me what was wrong, when the words poured out of my mouth like a streaming faucet. I spoke really fast and couldn't control myself. I just wanted so badly to get it out; to say everything before I changed my mind and lost my courage. I shivered in fear as I continued to spill out the horror that I had kept hidden far too long.

Within minutes, I realized I had blurted out the details of my abuse so quickly that it didn't come out exactly the way that I had rehearsed and planned. I looked up timidly to assess my mother's reaction. Her body was limp; she was staring at the wall. Her eyes were empty as she tried to make sense of what I had just told her. The facts had clearly hit her like a ton of bricks.

I will never forget the painful look of sadness in her eyes. It was a look that can only be compared to her hearing that someone had just died. I guess in a way…I had; or at least my innocence had died, and that fact filled her with sadness.

My mother wrapped her arms tightly around me, pulling me close to her as she tried to fight back the tears that welled up in her eyes. The sweet fragrance she always wore enveloped and comforted me as I melted in her arms, instantly feeling safe for the first time in a long time. She told me how sorry she was for all that I had been through, and how brave I had been for carrying the burden alone.

She continued to hold me and she listened closely as I told her all the horrible details of what had been happening to me. As I relived the abuse, the warmth of her body gave me the relief I had been yearning for. I was finally free from the dark secret that kept me in bondage way too long.

I felt not only relieved, but also very grateful when my mother assured me that what happened to me wasn't my fault at all. She added that we would confront my abuser together, as a family. Suddenly, all my fears about sharing my secret were gone. I felt lighter. The pressure cooker in my mind seemed to turn itself off. I did, however, convince my mother not to involve the police or anyone else. My family and I, like many other victims, chose to deal with the abuse ourselves and hope the pain would go away in time. Like other victims of abuse, we did not want to face ridicule or have to continue to relive what had happened. We just wanted to make sure it stopped, and by making it stop, we hoped the healing would begin.

My mother blamed herself for not protecting me better. I know that even to this day she still continues to carry that burden. I never told her how I'd already been molested two times before John, by two other men in Philadelphia; the last thing I wanted to do was overwhelm her with my history of abuse and molestation. She already carried guilt on her shoulders concerning John; I couldn't bear making that burden heavier by telling her about the others before him. Mainly, I just tried to reassure her that I was okay. That was my way of trying to ease her pain. As much as my mother assured me that what happened wasn't my fault, I still held on to my anger. I still blamed myself. The damage was done, and the negative opinions I had internalized were still there, deep inside me. I still questioned if they would ever go away.

Since the trauma that happened to me occurred at a young age, my life was literally shaped around the effects of the abuse. It completely took control of who I grew up to be. Most victims feel that they're at fault; I naturally thought that what happened to me on numerous occasions was something that I caused. Because I was too afraid and too ashamed to tell anyone what had happened to me, I grew up thinking that I was somehow a bad person who deserved, and maybe even asked for, what she got. I spent years blaming myself for being violated.

Children need to know that whatever they tell you, you will believe them, and that they are important to you. Secondly, educating children on "good touch" and "bad touch" at an early age is extremely important. It's important to empower children at an early age, and to teach them to use their voice if they feel that someone is violating them. I believe that teaching them to tell someone is vital in breaking the silence at an early age. Unfortunately, sexual predators usually are someone that we love and trust; so, if a loved one touches a child in the wrong way, it can be very confusing to the child. This is a life or death matter, and it is our responsibility to protect our children. We can do that through educating them and instilling a sense of trust in them that they can always come to us; that no matter what the situation is, we will always believe them and love them.

As a child…happiness was something that always seemed just beyond my reach. As an adult…the memories of being touched in all those very private places still haunted me. That was the reason that many nights, I lay awake in bed and cried myself to sleep. I would remember the tobacco smell on John's breath when he kissed me, and the dampness of his palms when he touched me in all those forbidden places. I knew the memories would continue to haunt me like deep scars; not even time could heal them.

I still wonder how things would have turned out if I had told my parents that I had been molested those summers while in Philly.

Would that have saved me from the horror I experienced with John, since sexual abuse was not a topic that was openly discussed during the time of my childhood years?

Unfortunately, I'll never know.

*****

As a little girl, I believed that when I got married and had a family, it would lead to a happy, fulfilling life. In real life, unfortunately, this belief proved itself wrong in a big way. I met Rick shortly after my eighteenth birthday. From his irresistible personality, great sense of humor, beautiful green eyes, and perfectly chiseled body, I thought that he was the answer to my prayers. I enjoyed our conversations so much that I did not realize how quickly time flew by when I was with him. Speaking to him made me feel like I had known him all my life. His friendly personality made me instantly feel comfortable with him.

After getting to know him better, I realized that I loved everything about him, especially when he would tell corny jokes to cheer me up when I was having a bad day. He also had a way of making me feel special when he would lean his tall framed body down so that he could kiss my forehead; he was so gentle and affectionate in that way. It didn't take long before we were inseparable. I couldn't wait to spend each and every day with him. I loved how protective he was over me; he had a way of making me feel safe. That was the reason I felt I could never get enough of him. I began to think of him as my knight in shining armor; enough so that I trusted him with my deepest, most shameful secret—my sexual molestation. Although he didn't receive the information as well as I had hoped he would, he did assure me that no matter what had happened to me in the past, he would never love me any less. That assurance helped me feel less like an outcast and more like a person. Our relationship was as close to perfect as any relationship could be, but it also had its ups and downs.

Rick struggled with the fact that his brother Elliot and I had a close friendship that started before Rick and I had gotten involved. He seemed extremely jealous, when ironically, if it had not been for Elliot, Rick and I would have never met. Yet Rick seemed to have a hard time letting go of the friendship Elliot and I still shared. I could see it in his eyes even as he continued to assure me he loved me. Soon it got hard to ignore the turbulence that was always there between us, hidden just beneath the surface. We began to break up and then get back together, over and over again. It was during one of those breakups that I found out I was pregnant with Rick's child. I called him the day after I found out, and we met that afternoon to discuss the pregnancy and make some plans. We decided to do the right thing for our baby, and get married. Back then, that is what people did when there was an unplanned pregnancy.

I expected the best—a happy marriage and a wonderful home for me and our baby on the way—as I took my vows while Rick slipped a ring on my finger. Surely, having a husband and a family would be enough to erase the painful memories that continued to haunt me; or at least I thought.

All our relationship problems seemed to vanish in the midst of our child's birth. The joy of bringing a new life into the world convinced us that our future would be nothing but perfect. Every day was an amazing adventure and our beautiful daughter, Shahnta enriched our lives profoundly as we watched her grow and thrive.

Unfortunately, the good times lasted less than a year before Rick's behavior began to change. As busy as the baby kept me, I could still see that he was preoccupied with something other than me and Shahnta. He was getting home later and later each night for one thing.

Had he found another woman? Was he having an affair? The thought would not leave my mind. I had to know the truth.

I spent a couple of days building up my courage before I finally confronted him one night. I even was more shocked when the answer he gave was not that there was another woman in his life, but that he had been out smoking crack cocaine with a co-worker every night. He didn't lie, or try to hide his drug use; he just told me matter-of-factly where he had been and what he had been doing. I had feared my husband was involved with another woman, but the truth was far worse; I knew crack cocaine was far more addictive than any personal relationship could ever be.

The first time Rick offered crack to me, he sat on the couch in our dimly lit living room holding a glass, genie-shaped pipe in his hands. I hadn't seen anything like it in person before, and I watched as he pulled smoke from the stem that stuck out of the glass pipe. I cursed at him when he offered it to me. My only knowledge of crack was the fact that Richard Pryor's face had caught on fire while free-basing cocaine. Seeing the images of Mr. Pryor's burn injuries all over the newspapers and TV and hearing the stories about how addicted he was, scared me enough to never want to try crack.

It wasn't that I had never done cocaine before—far from it. At the time, I was no saint when it came to the occasional snorting of co-caine, and I was fine with snorting it the way I always had. Rick felt that he and I had always been a team. So since he had discovered crack, he didn't want me to miss out on the euphoria of what taking that first hit of crack would feel like. Mistakenly viewing his willingness to share crack with me as a means of holding our marriage to-gether, it wasn't long before temptation got the best of me. I finally agreed and gave crack a try.

My husband was absorbed in the process of assembling the pipe carefully that night. He made sure every piece was put together as securely and perfectly as possible for my first hit. It was as if he was working on a major science project. I inhaled deeply on the pipe that night, taking all the smoke into my lungs. Within seconds, I was to-tally wrapped up in the feeling that I was floating on a gigantic pillow of clouds, a feeling that mesmerized me completely. Unfortunately, it lasted only about a minute—over with way too soon for my taste. At that point, I wanted to feel it again. I needed to feel it again.

The crack took control of our lives quickly; turning us against each other. The fact that we were spending so much money on our addiction soon resulted in the fact that we could no longer pay our rent, buy groceries, or pay our bills. We were high so much of the time that it resulted in our parents taking care of our little girl most of the time because we couldn't. It came as no surprise when we ended up separating later that year. We both believed that going our separate ways would help us address and deal with our addictions.

When I moved back to my parents' house, I was happy at the prospect of being able to stop smoking crack on my own. Rick, on the other hand, felt that he needed to go into rehab. I continued to support him as he completed his program, then we decided to move to California with one of his best friends. We believed, at that point, that if we re-moved ourselves from the people, places, and things that enabled us to use crack, then that would somehow remove the addiction from our lives. What we didn't realize then was that *we* were the people, places, and things that were causing us to use—and we were taking ourselves with us. It didn't take long for us to be back up to our old ways. We started smoking crack again just a few months after the move. Our new drug routine was ten times worse than before.

It wasn't long before we sent our daughter back to New Jersey with our families so that we could check ourselves into rehab—my first rehab experience. I prayed to God that by going to rehab I would be able to shake my addiction and finally have a normal life. With God's grace and support, I cleaned up my act and began attending twelve-step meetings faithfully and got a sponsor, as suggested by the rehab facility. At that point, my relationship with God had gotten stronger; I knew He loved me because He turned my life around. This motivated me to find a new way of life—one that could keep me clean. Getting clean was more of a struggle for Rick, but he was eventually able to get his life together too. I was clean but still not thinking clearly and decided that having another child would make all of our problems go away. Needless to say, it didn't work.

*****

I was seven months' pregnant when Rick was arrested on a drug-related charge. I remained supportive of him while he did his time in jail; after all, he was my husband—the father of my children. So, I made sure he knew I was behind him, even if he was in jail. It was rough, but I kept the lines of communication open, and gave him the encouragement of eventually having a life on the outside of prison walls.

Unfortunately, our efforts to make our marriage work proved impossible. Once outside of prison, Rick's desire to get high was in full throttle just like it had been before he went inside the concrete walls of the jail. Our desires to make the marriage work were not strong enough to overcome the reality that his drug addiction was still in the way.

I eventually had to surrender and let go of the marriage because I knew there was nothing more to be done to change things. The time we spent apart while he was in jail put a wedge between us, and even though we thought we could start off right where things had ended when he went in, we couldn't.

We have both moved on with our lives and now are different people. I am grateful we remain friends to this day, and have put the bad times and bad memories behind us.

Heartbroken because our marriage ended, I continued looking for love in all the wrong places, only to end up broken hearted once again. Soon after the divorce, I met Matthew; someone who I thought was my savior. I fell deeply in love with him so much so that I loved him more than myself. The attraction was so spontaneous, so strong, that I felt mesmerized. I knew the relationship was going to be serious as soon as we started dating, a few weeks later. Our connection was just as intense as our first encounter. It was obvious to me that although my marriage had wounded me deeply; somehow with Matthew in my life, I was ready to move on with my future.

I had been clean from cocaine for several years when I met Matthew, although I smoked marijuana occasionally, along with some social drinking while we were together. I felt okay with that, until Matthew and I started having knock out, drag out, fights. The stress, discomfort, and sadness caused me to go out to do the same thing I always did to comfort myself—I snorted cocaine.

I had shared my battle with cocaine addiction and my hidden secrets with Matthew early in our relationship. What I loved about him was that he never judged me. As our relationship came to a bitter end, I couldn't bear to tell him that my cocaine use had become as frequent as the fights we were having.

I was devastated when he left; broken-hearted from yet another failed relationship. Our relationship had ended so abruptly that it broke my heart, and I hadn't had time to heal. Although we continued to see each other periodically, I knew we would never be together again. I began to snort cocaine more and more often. Then, it was just a matter of time before I got the urge for something stronger—crack cocaine. I just didn't want to feel the pain anymore. The sadder and more depressed I felt, the more crack I smoked. The addiction had gotten the best of me again. My nights were filled with meeting my suppliers in seedy alleyways and abandoned buildings; always alone. I didn't seem to care about the danger I was putting myself in as I made attempts to score. Looking back, I know now that it was only God's grace that prevented me from getting raped or murdered.

My pain was so monumental that I felt like I could barely think at all.

One evening, while I was on my way to get high at a crack house in Newark, I found myself caught in the middle of a shoot-out. The fact that my only concern was how to get from my car to the crack house without being shot shows how totally out of touch I was with reality. Addiction was my jailer at that point. I truly, deeply believed I needed crack cocaine to survive, and unfortunately, put my life in jeopardy to get it.

I hated myself for what I had become; but I didn't have the will to surrender and let it go. If I had no idea that God was protecting me at the time, I know now that He most definitely made the difference between life and death for me back in those days. Drugs were the only way I had ever known to comfort myself and I hated myself for it. I felt abandoned—again—when Matthew left me. I continued to get high to block the pain of his rejection, even though I knew how quickly the drugs could destroy my life or even kill me.

Of all the possible consequences of my cocaine addiction, losing my children was the worst. It was a possibility that never failed to cause my chest to tighten and give me a dark, empty feeling in the pit of my stomach. Even though that possibility haunted me, it wasn't enough to bring me to the point where I was willing to stop getting high. At least not right away.

It hurt me deeply when my mother and sister took my children back with them to North Carolina. I knew it would be an abrupt and painful interruption in their young lives. It is always a hard transition for children to be uprooted from their home and their friends. Even worse, I knew the fact that they had to relocate was entirely my fault.

I found myself living in a personal hell at that point. I realized I needed to go back to rehab if I ever planned to get them back. I knew, suddenly, that only God could save me; I could never do it on my own.

Even though I wasn't sure what to do next, God took over and started the process for me. I fell into a deep depression about a week before my thirty-fifth birthday, and knew I needed professional help. I found a local psychiatrist in Summit, New Jersey who was willing to see me right away. My hope was that he would give me some kind of quick fix to instantaneously take away all the pain I was feeling.

The doctor suggested that I take a leave of absence from my job in order to give me time for the anti-depressants he was prescribing to work. I was happy at first when he prescribed not one, but three separate anti-depressants with instructions for me to take them together. He then added a fourth that he promised would provide immediate relief. It was a drug usually prescribed for psychosis and/or schizophrenia.

At the time, I was happy to have some relief from the pain, and I secretly expected the medications to lift me out of the pit I felt I was living in. But I soon found out that I was in for a surprise. The drugs made me feel lethargic to the point of not being able to function normally. Taking a shower in the morning and getting dressed required the effort of Hercules. I couldn't drive my car either because I felt drowsy all the time; so drowsy that it was not unusual for me to stay in bed all day.

It's hopeless! That's what I told myself that morning. *I need to end it all right now.* The thoughts were chanting over and over in my head. Suicide was suddenly a viable choice. I picked up a bottle of Codeine and I held the bottle tightly in my hands.

I'll take the whole bottle; take all the pills right now… the suicidal chanting began again.

I began to open the bottle until I realized I couldn't kill myself without saying good-bye to my daughters.

"A note—I'll write them a note!" I shouted out loud through tears which were streaming down my face as I went to get some paper and a pen. I sat back down, then holding the pen in one hand and the bottle of pills in the other. I tried to gather my thoughts through my drug haze. I put the bottle down and began the good-bye letter to my daughters:

My beloved daughters:

I want to tell you both how sorry I am for failing you as a mother. I love you both with all of my heart, and I am sorrier than words can ever say that I can't be here for you right now...

I looked at the words and suddenly, I knew that I couldn't keep going. It was better to just end it all right then. I took a deep breath for courage, then suddenly, I heard a voice deep inside me saying, *Hold on. Hold on just a little longer...*

Then I remembered Fair Oaks, a private psychiatric hospital and treatment center in Summit, New Jersey which specialized in drug and alcohol addiction. *If only they will admit me and let me stay there a few days, maybe I won't hurt myself;* my mind was still trying to rationalize my situation. As much as I felt like I wanted to die, I couldn't ignore the voice of God. He told me there was hope, and He urged me to keep going.

I forced myself to look up the hospital's number and make the call. The woman who answered spoke softly and sounded nice, that helped me continue taking the steps I needed to take in order to survive. When she asked me my name, I told her and I also informed her of my plans to end my life by swallowing the bottle of pills. She listened closely and then told me how Fair Oaks could help me.

As she continued questioning me in a very caring manner, I found myself laying the bottle of pills down and willingly answering her questions. First, I told her about my cocaine addiction, and then I gave her my medical insurance information. After twenty minutes on the phone, she told me there was a bed available; I could have it, if I got there ASAP. I agreed to do so. After all, I knew my life depended on it. I felt a little bit of relief and was hopeful that I would finally get the help I needed. I quickly threw some clothes in a bag and jumped in my car.

By the grace of God, I still had my sanity. I went to the facility and checked myself in, and after a day of being on the psychiatric ward, I proceeded to check myself out. I was informed by the ward nurse that there was a 72-hour clause on the admittance sheet that I had signed. I had only been there almost 48 hours at that point; not long, but long enough for me to take a good look at my life from a new and different point of view. It was also long enough to jolt me into a new reality and remind me how far I had really come on my life journey.

I realized right then and there that if I could somehow manage to cling to just a little bit of hope, it might be possible for me to turn my life around. I thought back to what my cousin, Ferrell, had suggested about reading the Hebrews' scripture in the Bible. I decided to try *faith* – the strongest faith I'd ever possessed – to turn my life around.

My Fair Oaks experience had been invaluable in giving me a whole new perspective on my life and willingness to put my trust in God. The opportunity to do that presented itself quickly when some-one suggested that I attend a revival at Fountain Baptist, a local church in Summit. Ironically, it wasn't far from Fair Oaks. I was pleasantly surprised when I attended the revival. The hope and spirit that surrounded me there made me go home feeling much better about my life.

On the third day of the revival, a young pastor gave a testimony about how he had turned his life over to Christ. His sermon filled me with so much hope that I knew that I, too, was ready to turn my life over to Christ. Everything I had been through had given me the chance to see how God helped pull me through some trying times, and some rather destructive behaviors. It was His love that kept me. I knew that my decision to turn my will and my life over to His care would be one of the best decisions I had ever made.

Suddenly my world changed. I got up one morning and knew I couldn't endure another day of hurting myself and living a double life. Trying to appear normal during the day and getting high at night had become much too hard to maintain. Getting my hands on drugs every day was yet another problem. It had never been easy, but it was getting harder every day.

What little faith I had before I started using, the drugs had already taken that from me. Cocaine had been my God—my only God—far longer than I wanted to admit. Like an epiphany of deliverance, the day arrived when I realized I couldn't continue down the road I knew would eventually cost me my life.

However, the day of my epiphany was different. I had come to the deep and definite realization that determination alone was not enough to keep me clean. God was the only one who could guide me as I journeyed deep inside my heart to find and address the issues that had kept me in pain, and which threatened to take everything: my children, my job, and my life itself.

I knew learning how to love myself would be the toughest battle of my life, but with God in my heart, always with me, I felt ready to try.

That night, I got on my knees and lifted my hands to the heavens. I prayed to God to remove my drug obsession and end my sick, desperate need to get high. I held my hands high as a sign of humble surrender to show God how serious I was as I let the tears stream down my face uncontrollably. An undeniable sense of peace and calm quickly came over me. I took that as a sign of God's confirmation that He had heard me. My tears turned into sobs even as I praised God. Suddenly, I knew I was going to be okay.

I began to take a long look at my childhood; something I knew I needed to do in order to start my healing journey. My childhood, after all, was the time when the seeds of my wounds had first been planted. Those seeds blossomed into self-destructive habits which soon became comfortable for me because in the deepest place of my heart, I didn't feel worthy of my existence

I've spent a large portion of my life mentally checking out from reality in an attempt to avoid the pain of my past; not to mention, trying to escape the voices in my head that were repeatedly trying to convince me that I was worthless. My behavior was typical of someone like me – a victim of non-consensual sexual violence. Moments of violation can linger long after perpetration; and sexual abuse can have damning effects on its victims. It is not uncommon for victims to unknowingly believe that they are responsible for the infliction of the abuse. There can be a constant struggle going on inside of them which makes them question their self-worth and their actions leading up to the abuse. Because of this, lives are being destroyed, leaving lifelong wounds that may never heal. That's why I struggled through life, allowing my circumstances to have their way with me – dictating my every thought, every feeling, every move, and every decision.

As I began to walk with Christ, I came to the realization that you must love yourself before you can love anyone else. I had been so desperate to fill the spiritual void inside of me that I had tried to heal the wound instantly by putting a Band-Aid on it, instead of doing the work it would really take to heal the old internal wounds. At the same time, I had a need for someone else to love me because I didn't know how to love myself. I looked for that love in every relationship and then wondered why they never worked. My repeated attempts at putting a Band-Aid over a gaping wound was futile.

In my case, God had to get my attention in order for me to trust in Him and His powers. Facing storms, then being rescued by God, strengthened my faith immeasurably. God showed me, every day of my life, how He was there for me. Now, years later, I can clearly see how much He loves me rather than regarding the events of my life as coincidences as I had in the past.

I know now that every storm life presents us with is an opportunity for us to practice our faith. *How can we have a testimony if we don't first have a test?* God is always working on something far greater and better for our lives than anything we can ever imagine. We must be patient and allow the miracles to unfold.

God's plan for me is, and has always been, perfect. Unfortunately, I couldn't understand that plan and how it was going to work until I was thoroughly convinced while doing my usual morning prayer. I heard Him speak to me. Tears of gratitude and joy streamed down my face as I prayed; I could feel His presence in my room. Warmth suffused my body as He very clearly told me He wanted me to minister to others. If God wanted to use me to tell my story to help others heal, then I knew it was mandatory for me to heal first.

I began my search to find a therapist who could help me face my fears and move beyond the scars of sexual abuse. It was very important for me during my healing process to find someone I could trust and be totally honest with. I needed to feel safe before I could open up and reveal all of my deepest and darkest secrets. It took time to build a trusting relationship.

I found the right therapist to help me. I felt completely comfortable with Nan, and knew that I had finally found a therapist whom I could completely trust. Her warm and caring personality made it easy for me to let down the walls I had built up for years. I was finally able to tell her about every aspect of my sexual molestation.

*****

Before I began to work with Nan, I knew my drug addiction had always gotten in the way, taking precedence over the real reason I went to therapy. In terms of my relationships with therapists, I had used my drug addiction and depression as a smoke screen. It allowed me to avoid thoroughly facing my sexual molestation, and the ways in which it had damaged me. The more I talked with Nan about the abuse and was able to accept my feelings, the easier therapy became.

Healing is a very personal and unique experience; every person finds solace at his or her own individual pace. What may be beneficial for one person may not be the remedy for another.

The most important thing I learned during my therapy sessions was about forgiveness. The first person I needed to forgive was me. Forgiving others is hard. It entails us stepping outside of our hurts and fears long enough to be Godlike in our behavior. That's hard to do; but if we have any sort of relationship with God, we find a way to own a spirit of forgiveness. Sometimes we do that with the caveat of, "Forgiving, but not forgetting." Even if we choose not to forget, somehow, because of the influence of God, we find a way to forgive others.

However, we are not as lenient on ourselves.

It is much harder for us to extend that same spirit of forgiveness toward ourselves for the abuse we inflict inward. We have a tendency to be harder on our own actions, or lack thereof, than we are concerning the actions of others.

In my own circumstances, I realized that I was very angry at my abusers, but I always found ways to make excuses for what they did to me. This was subconscious on my part, but I thought by minimizing what happened, I could fool myself into thinking that I wasn't as hurt as I was. Only with the passage of time, and a deep glance at how I was carrying the anger around like a chip on my shoulder, was I able to lighten my emotional load. Once I did, I was able to forgive my attackers. But that release did not include the blame I placed on myself. Somehow, although I did not know I was doing it, I had somehow forgiven them and shifted the blame from them to me.

I was angry with myself, and resentful concerning the sexual abuse for most of my life. It was an inner hatred that I could not shake for a very long time. Much more importantly, I truly and deeply believed that I had done something to cause the abuse to happen to me. I felt like I had a neon sign on my forehead that lit up as an advertisement requesting abusers to use me at will. I did not realize, until I went through therapy, that I was not responsible for what my abusers had done to me. Their sins were not mine to bear. Nothing I had said or done warranted me being used and abused. It was a long journey to get to that place of fruition and acceptance.

I found, along my journey of self-forgiveness, that many victims feel guilty and ashamed when abuse happens to them. They carry the guilt that something they did had to have been an instigator of their torment and pain. Victims fail to realize that predators don't need provocation; their need to prey on the weak and innocent is fuel enough.

If you are the victim of abuse, the most important thing for you to remember is this: it is not your fault! By defining yourself as the cause, you are minimizing the fact that what happened to you is a casualty. You cannot, and should not, take ownership of someone else's actions. In committing the act of abuse, the perpetrator wanted to take your power; don't continue to let them have it by owning their sins as your own. You must stop the cycle of power through abuse, and that begins by forgiving yourself and realizing that you are not to blame. Only then can you learn how to nurture the wounded child inside of you, as I did.

Thinking back to my own abuse still haunts me. Only with the help of God have I been able to move forward beyond the abuse, and beyond the pain. I continue to pray for my abusers, realizing that they need God's help just as much as I do, and I'm always careful not to wish them any harm. They are lost souls that need guidance, and the spirit of forgiveness has shown me not to desire vengeance for my pain.

At one point in my therapy, I decided to confront one of my abusers. The courage I had to muster to tell him how negatively he had impacted my life was very therapeutic for me. I needed to feel the sense of power in stepping from behind my shame and putting the blame where it belonged   in his lap. Although I knew the confrontation wouldn't change the past, and what had happened, it was very empowering and definitely helped me in moving the healing process forward.

Confronting my abuser was also an opportunity for me to stand up for myself as an adult, dissipating some of the pain that resulted from the fact that I could not stand up for myself as a child. There was an extreme sense of gratification in that role reversal. I also needed the confrontation in order to give myself permission to fully forgive my abuser.

I knew it was time to clear out and remove the anger and bitterness that were festering inside me. A feeling I like to compare to having high cholesterol. Cholesterol blocks our arteries, preventing blood from pumping freely to our hearts and through our bodies. Anger felt the same way to me; it kept me stuck in the same place and blocked me from growing and loving. My anger harmed me much more than the abusers whom I had convinced myself I would always hate. The lingering feeling hurt me more than the person had.

I also knew that part of my journey to healing included a need for me to forgive my parents. As a teen, misguided in my feelings and not knowing where to turn, I was angry with them for not being able to see the signs that I had been abused. I was even angrier with them for not realizing that my drug use and destructive behavior all stemmed from the abuse. I harbored a sense of resentment that they could not see past the walls I had built up. It was because I found a way to disguise the source of my pain. That feeling hung around my neck like an expensive silk tie of blame.

Later in life, as part of my therapy and healing process, I made the decision to talk to my parents about my trauma and my feelings toward both of them. It was a powerful step that helped us all to begin healing. The unspoken demon was finally slayed.

Most people don't recognize the fact that victims are not the only ones harmed by abuse. Many parents, who learn that their children have been abused, suffered a great deal of anger, emotional pain, and guilt as well. Most of the time, the family, as a whole, suffers in shame. The abuse becomes a dirty little secret kept in the hall closet, out of sight of others. Everyone involved feels that they are the cause or source of its conception. In fact, it is not uncommon for parents of abused children to beat themselves up emotionally for years. They feel they did not protect their child in a manner that would never have left them vulnerable to the abuse in the first place. Sometimes parents blame themselves more than they blame the perpetrator for what happened.

When confronted with sexual molestation, some families prefer to keep their problems inside of their homes. They falsely believe that outside help is not needed, and that family unity will be enough to ease and erase all of the pain. I now know that the whole family unit can benefit from professional counseling if they participate in it together. Once a family can articulate in their own words and actions that the unthinkable has actually happened in their family, then and only then, can the bond of family unity conquer all. Counseling helps each member to heal, and be freed from their own individual, self-imposed guilt and shame.

Having put the chore of forgiving my abuser, myself, and my parents behind me, I had one more obstacle to tackle in order to fully address this process. The last, but rather critically important thing I had to face and forgive myself for was the trauma I had put my children through. They were the silent victims in the trickle-down effect of my abuse as a child. Sometimes we have to remove the rose-colored glasses of denial and just accept things as they are or were, and take steps accordingly toward corrective action.

I will never be able to get those years in my daughters' lives back. I am glad to say that I've also accepted the message from God of how forgiving children can be by nature. There is nothing more wonderful than the unconditional love for a parent given by a child. That message echoes from our love of our Heavenly Father to spilling over into our own personal relationships with our own children. A child's love is unconditional and has no boundaries. For that, I am truly grateful. My daughters love me, respect me, and are proud of me, despite all the mistakes I've made along the way. My mistakes and irresponsible choices made their lives harder than what it should have been. They never used it against me, or as sources of ridicule or retaliation. Their pride and love are the best and the most rewarding gifts of all.

The gifts, in the form of my daughters' unconditional love and pride in me, were just what I needed in order to start looking at myself differently. I began giving myself the same unconditional love that I received from them. I began to feel an inner peace and self-love having explored the issues that resulted from my abuse. A trained therapist helped me to deflate the air in the balloon cycle of abuse that was my life, and potentially theirs. My new feelings about myself became the helium to a new balloon of a life cycle for all of us to follow. Their love helped us break a vicious cycle. We were able to start anew and build upon a foundation of understanding and persevering in spite of. Forgiving yourself also opens the doors to creating healthy relationships. God has given me a second chance in marriage. He has blessed me with a supportive and loving husband who accepts me for the person that I am. I first had to learn to love myself before I could truly love someone else in a healthy way.

The lesson I learned during my journey to forgiveness was simple, yet profound. I found out that only when we forgive others, as well as ourselves completely, are we able move on with our lives. It allows our hearts to receive all the blessings and love that God has waiting for us.

Today, I work through my past by practicing positive affirmations instead of beating myself up. I am more health conscious, and I now accept myself for who I am. I am furthering my education, and I practice being the best person that I can be each day. I no longer have to self-medicate myself to numb my pain. I've worked through the pain and have forgiven myself for what I thought was my fault. I have forgiven those who have violated me because I know that holding on to the anger will only destroy me. The shackles of my shame have been removed and I am now free. Free from thinking that I was a bad person, and free from thinking that all I would ever be is damaged goods. Today, I know that I am worth so much more, and that I am blessed and highly favored.

With all the contentment I've had, the traces of the sad little girl I was, and of the sexual abuse I endured, still lingers. Some days are better than others; but no matter what, regardless of how far I've come, there are some wounds that will still take a lifetime to heal. Through counseling, education, and research, I learned that if sexual abuse happens at an early age and the right steps are taken, there is a good chance that the victim can begin healing and live a healthy life. Survival has no purpose if it is not used to elevate others from their pain.

We can't run from our demons; God wants us to address them and be triumphant over them. When God is satisfied that we've learned the lesson we were supposed to learn, that is when He will allow us to move forward. I will continue on my personal healing journey and share my story in an attempt to be an advocate for abuse victims everywhere. I have learned that no matter the nature and depth of the struggle, no matter how many lessons I need to learn, I can always count on God to do His work. I, like so many abuse victims, am a work in progress.

In my case, He continues to use me to uplift others. My life story of battling with drug addiction, failed relationships, and depression is clearly a direct result of how God can turn things around. From the pits of being in crack houses and losing my children, to being an advocate for victims everywhere…God uses me. I had to reach the realization that I would have no inner peace until I learned to love myself unconditionally; the way that He does. It took all that I went through for me to understand that true beauty lies not on the outside, but deep within. My exterior body is just the shell that holds my authentic self.

I also know now that healing is not a destination, but a journey. There will never be an end to how we heal; it is an ongoing existence that we go through one day at a time. As long as I walk with God, and continue to do His will, I will continue to heal – every day of my life. There is peace in knowing that God will always be with me as long as I have faith.

I pray that this book reaches the hands of every little girl, boy, man, and woman whose life may have been touched by any kind of abuse. In sharing my story, and the stories of other courageous survivors, I hope you may never have to suffer as we have. If you believe that you have ever been violated, I urge you to find someone you can trust and talk to them so that you can begin your own healing journey.

In conclusion, I would like to say that whether you are a victim of abuse or not, we are all battling something in our lives. We all suffer, in some form or fashion, with something that wants to control us or define who we are. Being vulnerable is part of being human. God can show you the way to heal from self-destructive behaviors and feelings; all you need to do is open your heart in order to receive Him.

Part II

We Are Not Alone - Other Victims Speak

A Glimpse at a Detoured Life

The events that children experience during childhood have a way of shaping them into the adults they will become. Whether the events are good or bad, those experiences will either reinforce good self-esteem or destroy it. Specifically, children who have experienced traumatic events such as child sexual abuse are robbed early of the opportunity to have positive self-esteem. The chances of feeling good about themselves, or becoming the person they dreamed of, are destroyed.

In many cases, children don't tell what happened to them; the abuse becomes a life-long secret. If they do not receive early treatment, chances are they will not become healthy adults. The shame, pain, and guilt can lead them to a place of darkness and undesirable lifestyles in order to cope. Although in some cases, victims will submerge themselves in positive activities to disassociate from the abuse. Unfortunately, the memories of the abuse will tend to resurface at some point in their lives.

Tragically, there are victims who are so deeply wounded that they have drastically taken measures into their own hands to make the pain stop. For example, the tragic story of Stacey Lannert, who suffered terrifying abuse at the hands of her alcoholic father for ten years. At the age of eighteen, Stacey shot and killed her father. As a little girl, she was told by her father that her mother knew about the abuse, but didn't care. This was his way of keeping Stacey silent, and she never told a soul. Instead, Stacey threw herself into excelling in sports and other academic activities as a way to cope with the abuse.

However, when Stacey realized her father was turning his attention toward her younger sister, who was on the verge of becoming his next victim, Stacey shot and killed her father. Stacey was found guilty of first-degree murder and sentenced to life in prison without the possibility of early release. After spending decades behind bars, never giving up on herself, the history of her abuse was revealed. Finally, she received clemency and was freed from prison after eighteen years.

In recent years, there are more women in prison than any other time in American history. Many of these women have been victims of physical, mental, and sexual abuse. Child sexual abuse has a way of derailing a victim's life, leading them to destructive lifestyles. Many of the women who are incarcerated, I am sure, never planned to end up there. Circumstances have a way of shaping and detouring a person's life. Child sexual abuse is no different and causes so much harm; if untreated, it causes a lifetime of unhealed scars. Post-Traumatic Stress Disorder (PTSD), depression, drug and alcohol addiction, prostitution, teen suicide, and teen pregnancy are only some of the effects of sexual abuse. There is so much shame and pain involved, that the victims seek comfort wherever they can find it. Unfortunately, some of the coping mechanisms lead to lifestyles that have a snowball effect in the wrong direction. Because a person may engage in something that is bad does not make them a bad person.

A recent study has shown that an astounding number of incarcerated women are victims of childhood sexual abuse. Studies suggest that between 47 and 82 percent of women have endured that crime. Other studies say 94 percent of incarcerated women have been victimized sexually; some as children, others as adults. Abuse clearly destroys lives, and there are women whose stories have been overlooked and swept away. Marvella's story is a depiction of an innocent child who was robbed of her childhood and was never given the opportunity to heal. Those wounds detoured her life to a place that has changed it forever. My hope is that her traumatic story will shed light on this epidemic and bring our society out of darkness. I will continue fighting for Marvella, and the many victims like her who are incarcerated and deserve a second chance.

Chapter Two
A Detoured Life: Marvella's Story

L ife has its own way of molding and shaping us; at least that is what it has done for me. I know I have been transformed into a different person than I was fourteen and a half years ago. I am not the same quiet, shy, vulnerable woman that I once was; the one who was subject to all kinds of abuse. Mentally, I'm stronger now. I can talk openly about my pain and suffering without associating it with any inner guilt or shame. I can now forgive others; not only that, but I can receive forgiveness from others and from myself as well. I am at peace with myself; a task that took a long time for me to accomplish.

I've grown in a lot of ways – working on myself from the time I stepped foot onto this ground. Plain and simple, I'm a caged bird. It's not the perfect place to be to say the least, but it's where my life's journey has led me. I realize that I am a product of my circumstances; some of which were the result of the actions of others, and some of which were self-imposed. All have shaped and molded me into who I am today.

The first domestic violence group I attended was in 2004 or 2005. I was so wound up at the time; a broken existence of a woman. I had so many hurts, habits, and hang-ups. Mentally shattered, I never really talked to anyone at those group meetings. All I could do was listen and wait; hoping that one day, the stories, the encouragement, and the support I received would take hold long enough for me to be able to let my voice be heard. It was a hard and long road I had to travel to get to where I am now. Over the years, I have participated in numerous domestic violence and self-help groups. Each one slowly chipped away at the wall I had built up. Eventually, they helped me to become the woman that I am today.

I have begun to realize that every day there's something new to learn; good or bad. No matter the hurt, pain, or obstacles...you live and learn. Having been touched by the things in life that I have been touched by, I know I am forever changed. I am a different person. I have a better understanding of life and the women around me now. I have great compassion for the women who are still suffering and hurting from the same kind of events that caused me heartache and pain. Their struggle is real, just like mine was; but theirs is ongoing. My heart cries out for them.

Don't get me wrong, I have always had compassion and love for others; even regarding what others may say about me personally. It's just that now, I have both sympathy and empathy for women like me; women who fell victim to molestation and abuse as if it were a normal part of life. When that way of living was my norm, I did not know how to show my compassion or sisterhood with them; I was too busy trying to get by and make it from day to day to care about anyone else's personal hell. I couldn't cry for them, or with them, because my voice had been silenced by my own shame. I realize now that there is no shame in being a victim. The shame is in remaining one.

I've made some drastic changes from the person I was fourteen and a half years ago. I now understand all that happened to me, and why I had to travel that long hard road. While I will never forget, today I can forgive. While I can't get back the days, months, and years of innocence that were taken from me...today I can take time for myself. And while I may not be loveable in the eyes of others, today I can love me.

*****

The Little Girl Who Never Grew Up

My memories of my childhood are a mixture of what I remember, and what was told to me by my siblings. Admittedly, I blocked out a lot; simply because there were some things I didn't ever want to remember. They were too painful. Other events made sure they had a home in my memory bank, whether I wanted them there or not.

From a very young age, I was moved from foster home to foster home. My mother died when I was seven years old. The little time I spent with her was not good at all; at least as far back as my memory goes. All I remember about my upbringing with my mother is that there was a lot of fighting, drinking, arguing, and crying. Those were the elements that were a part of my daily life in my mother's home, and none of which were a place for a young, impressionable child. Maybe that is why my mother didn't fight to keep me or my siblings with her. I'm not sure if my mother's unstable household was a factor for her or not, or if it was just the fact that she really didn't care one way or the other about her children. The sad part is that I will never know.

The first foster home I was placed in was okay, except for the fact that I was never really allowed to spend time with my real family. Most of my siblings were spread out in other foster care homes throughout the state. While I was in that first foster home, my mother and two of my sisters passed away. By the time I was eight years old, I was moved to another home. I didn't like it there. The lady was mean, and her husband was quiet; they were older people with very little patience for children. The woman hit me in the head once because I wet the bed. She beat me out of my sleep for it, and there was blood everywhere.

That event was one of the first horrible things that happened to me; the key word being "one." The couple had five sons; all of them were married. The sons didn't come around much, but there was one man – a friend of the family – who did. I'm not sure how often he visited my foster parents before I came to live with them, but he was there all the time once I moved in, and he molested me every chance that he got. That "friend" of the family was overly friendly with me. So there I was…this little girl, terrified, and living in fear, being molested, afraid to tell, and afraid to talk.

My mother had twelve kids; of those children, my sister Beverly was the only one who actually stayed with our mother to the very end. I was seven and Beverly was fourteen when our mother put me and the rest of my siblings in foster care. Mother never even bothered to try to place Beverly in foster care because Beverley had a job as a babysitter at the time, so she had been bringing money into the home since the age of eleven. That saved her from foster care – a fate the rest of us had no choice but to endure; besides, my mother knew that Beverly wouldn't go even if she tried to make her.

Beverly would later tell me that our mother was a drunk and unable to care for her children. At the time, five of my siblings and I went into foster care because our family was facing eviction from our home. Beverly refused to go into foster care, and she stayed with our mother in Philly. Two of my older siblings – Irma Jean and Robert – were in and out of the house at the time, and sometimes they lived with Beverly and my mother after the rest of us were sent off. There was another brother by the name of William, but none of us ever met him. He had been given away as an infant and was not in the family home with the other younger children.

I learned from Beverly that she and William had both initially been given away. Our mother had rheumatic fever at one time, and she had given William away to a couple of different women to care for him until she got better. When our mother got better and came back for her child, the woman who had him at the time demanded $500 for the cost of his care. My mother did not have the money to pay the amount that was demanded, so she just left William with the woman who had been caring for him during her illness.

Beverly indicated that she never saw our brother William again until mother's funeral in 1969. One of our cousins found him living in Millville, and they brought him to our mother's funeral. Since William had been taken away when he was five months old, mother's funeral was the first time he had seen her, or had a chance to meet his brothers and sisters.

Shortly after we were put in foster care, my sister Loretta and my sister Yolanda both ran away from their foster homes and they made their way to Philly. Somehow they found our mother. The two of them stayed with Beverly and our mother; she never sent them back to their foster homes, and they lived with her for approximately three years before our mother died of an aneurysm. The children that remained in foster care, including me, were allowed to attend our mother's funeral. It's a sad reality that our mother's funeral was the first chance that some of her children had a chance to get to know one another, or to even see each other in years.

My sisters and I have always been very bitter about being placed in foster care. The four of us were there for ten years. Our mother did not visit any of us at all during that time. For a short period of time, my sister Yvette and I lived in the same foster home. On one occasion, our older sisters Beverly and Yvonne came to the foster home to bring a cake to Yvette for her birthday. The foster care parents accepted the cake, but they would not let our sisters visit us because they said that Yvette and I were too young. I was eight and Yvette was ten at the time. We were young, that's true; but we were not too young to spend time with our family. My time in foster care had a way of distancing me, literally and figuratively, from my real family. I felt very little of a connection to them because I was moved around so much, and my time to be around them was very limited. In 1973, my sister Yvonne was stabbed forty-four times. She died at the age of nineteen, and I didn't attend the funeral.

Death and separation seemed to go hand and hand within my family, and I was becoming numb to both. When I was about fifteen years old, the father of my two younger sisters died. Their aunts came from Florida and signed all three of us out of foster care. Even though they took me with them, I felt that I was not wanted by them because they were not my real aunts. I didn't feel love from them; just obligation. I didn't want to be anyone's charity case, so when we were at the Philadelphia train station, I looked at them and said, "I don't want to go." They couldn't get into their pocketbooks fast enough. They put me in a cab, and I never saw my sisters again. That was over thirty-five years ago.

I don't remember exactly how I came to live in New Jersey after getting out of foster care. I think it was because my sister Beverly was there for a while when she was pregnant, and I went there with her. Anyway, somehow, by the age of sixteen, I ended up living with members of my father's family. I was very excited. At last, for the first time in a long time, I was with my real family – my blood. That excitement was short lived though. I don't think I was in New Jersey a year when my first cousin raped me in my sleep. It turned out that being with my real blood didn't mean that I would be protected or loved. Quite the contrary; real blood gave me the same real abuse that I received in foster care, and somehow, that was worse to me. To top it off, my father's family covered it all up; and even to this day, they don't speak about it.

Whatever is covered up will be uncovered, and every secret will be made known; so then, whatever you have said in the dark will be heard in broad daylight. Luke 12:2-3

By the time I was eighteen, I was a bonafide alcoholic. I had been drinking heavily during my teens, trying to erase the pain and silence the hurt inside me; it became worse by the time I was in my twenties. The mind is an interesting mechanism; things that bother us mentally have a way of affecting us physically. I was ill a lot growing up, and I also suffered from deep emotional problems. There was always something wrong with me and I had a lot of problems with my stomach. I found it hard to keep a job. My mind and body were attacking me at every turn. Others often told me that I always appeared as if I had "Something on my mind." Little did they know…I did have things on my mind. Secret things. Horrible things. The only time I seemed to be happy or at peace with myself was when I was drunk. That was the only time my mind wasn't screaming for help.

Once, Beverly asked me why I drank so much. I looked at her and replied, "Ever since he raped me, I just don't give a shit about myself or anything else!"

Making that statement was the first time that I allowed the little girl inside me to have her say. Even though I had aged from the time I was first sent away to foster homes by my mother, I was still a little girl inside who – due to sexual abuse – had never really had a chance to grow up.

*****

Parental Units

When I think back over the sources of my depression, the fact that I was never ever able to get pregnant comes to mind. Secretly, I wanted to have kids to right all the wrongs that I felt were done to me. I always felt that if I had a normal upbringing and had been part of a two-parent home, maybe my life would have been easier and I wouldn't have been subjected to such pain and abuse. In my mind, I wanted a do-over in the form of fixing things by having my own children and giving them the love, normalcy, and protection that I never got. But as fate would have it, I never got that chance, and the reality of that has always haunted me.

In addition to being an alcoholic, my mother was in and out of the hospital all the time. Some of those instances were at the hands of my father. He was married to my mother and had a woman on the side. I was not the only child that my parents had together. My father was the father of six of the twelve children that my mother gave birth to. He not only planted his seed with my mother, but he also had four children with his other women. Three of those children are now deceased, and the fourth is serving a life sentence in prison.

Although it has never been addressed or acknowledged, Beverly also believed that my father was the father of my oldest sister's first child. Taboo topics always seem to be swept under the rug in our family, so I was never able to get validation of that; but Beverly stated that she had caught my father having sex with our sister several times, and that each of them gave her money not to tell anyone. My oldest sister was not my father's child by birth, but she was his daughter by circumstance. As much as I cared for my father, I believe Beverly. I also believe that my father is the father of his own step-grandchild; sick as that may sound.

My father also used to beat up on my mother a lot when they were together. Once, he shoved her down a flight of stairs as me and my siblings in the house looked on. Because of the beating my mother received, she ended up losing the baby she was carrying at the time. That was the second child that my mother lost due to my father's beatings. As the story goes, when I was a baby, my father hit my mother in the head with a hatchet, and she ended up hospitalized for a while. My father left to tend to his other family, and my oldest sister took care of her siblings while our mother was in the hospital. With no food in the house at the time, our sister fed us dog food. When our neighbors learned of our circumstances, they contacted our aunts to let them know what was going on while our mother was away. In a normal family, if aunts would have learned of the condition their sister's children were in, they would step in and take care of their nieces and nephews. That didn't happen in our case. Instead, our aunts contacted DYFS, and all of my mother's children who lived in the house were place in DYFS's care until our mother was released from the hospital.

After my mother was released from the hospital, my father continued to come around when he felt like it, and when it was comfortable for his two-family lifestyle. He also continued to beat on my mother at will. Eventually, my mother got tired of playing second to my father's other women, and she met a new man and took up with him.

For a while, the new man treated my mother well, and he ended up fathering two more children with my mom. But soon that relationship became ugly as well, and he tried to beat up on my mom as well. There was a problem with his evil intentions. By the time he had entered my mom's life, most of her children were older. It wasn't as easy for any man to put their hands on her because her children were there to defend her.

After my mom's children beat up our mother's new boyfriend, he left our mother and ended up marrying another woman. My mother met another man about a year later, and she ended up marrying him. By this time, my mother was done having children so none were born from the union of her and her new husband. However, as if there was a neon sign on her head that she was a punching bag for men, the beatings continued with the new man in my mother's life. My sisters saw our stepfather beating our mother, and the two of them confronted the man and beat him up. The police were called, and my oldest sister, not Beverly, was arrested for cutting him several times. The beating served as a warning for my stepfather. He never hit my mother again.

My mother, my siblings and I, never really had anyone to help any of us out; we were victims of our circumstances for all of our lives. Tragedy, hurt, pain, suffering, and ultimately death followed our family for years. My mother died at the age of forty-three from an aneurysm, and one of my sisters died of the same malady at the age of thirty. Another one of my sisters died at twenty-nine of uterine cancer, and one was stabbed to death at nineteen. One of my brothers spent fourteen months in a coma after being mugged, eventually our oldest brother gave consent to disconnect his life support; he died two weeks later at the age of twenty-eight. My oldest brother who gave the consent died at fifty-two of esophageal cancer.

I don't believe in curses; but if I did, I would swear that there was a curse on my mother and the fruit of her womb. My mother and all of her children had it rough, in one way or another; some more so than the others.

*****

Life goes on

I came to believe that a power greater than myself could restore me to sanity. Step 2.

From the dark place that was my humble beginning, I was moved to another home and then another. Altogether, I spent ten years in foster care. I was one of twelve children born to my mother; but six are deceased, and I also have four half sisters and brothers. Of those four stepsiblings, three of them are deceased. I had seen so much death by the time I was in my twenties, that I started to worry about my own life.

My mother had three sets of children by three different men; but it should be noted that I was not the only one in the family who was molested. It was relayed in later years, that my two younger sisters were molested while in foster care as well. Hearing their stories triggered something inside of me. It made me remember the extent of my own abuse.

In one foster home, I told my foster mother that her friend was molesting me. I hoped that by telling her, I would get some relief and help for my situation. Instead of confronting her friend about his actions, the woman cracked me over the head with a shoe. I never got stitches to close the wound. It also began a cycle within me of remaining silent when it came to me being abused.

A few years later, I finally got a chance to meet my father's family, only for it to turn into a case of being ostracized, to some degree, because I revealed being raped by my cousin while I was sleeping in bed with his children. No one in my father's family gave any comfort or credence to the assault. They kept it hush hush, and hoped the nightmarish memory of it would just go away. They were more interested in protecting my cousin from prosecution than they were in dealing with what happened to me – the person who was viewed as the "newcomer to the family." That incident, just like the other, seemed to instill in me a sense that speaking of my abuse only made matters worse. It seemed like suffering in silence was the only answer.

With the second incidence of being raped in my sleep, I became angry, bitter, enraged, and very unhappy. I was so blind that I couldn't see anything but darkness. I felt I had to get away in order to survive. So, I left the family that I thought would show me love because I was their blood. I felt I had no option but to leave. It seemed as though no one liked me, or even cared about me. Everyone seemed mad at me for speaking about the unthinkable things that were being done to me. In their eyes, I wasn't a victim; I was a traitor because I spoke up about the abuse. Since I couldn't live in silence, and I couldn't stand the look in their eyes every time I was around them, I left. I went to the streets, and I lived with anyone that would take me in. I had no idea what would be ahead of me, but I felt I had no other option if I wanted to avoid more mental and sexual abuse.

Satan, who is the God of this world, has blinded the minds of those who don't believe. They are unable to see the glorious light of the good news. 2 Corinthians 4:4

I was sixteen years old and living on the streets. I was in school, but I dropped out soon after the rape. It was the best option for me because I had no structure, no family foundation, I really didn't have a place to live, and I was not able to concentrate on going to school anyway. My mind was not focused on learning anything.

At the time, I had a friend who had a big family. I began to hang out with her family a lot, and at one point, her mother told me that she loved me as if I was one of her very own children. My heart was overjoyed. That was all that I ever wanted to hear—that I was LOVED!!!! I had never heard that word before. I didn't know what love was, but I knew I wanted to feel it.

As I spent more and more time at my friend's house and began doing more things with her family, I soon started going out with my friend's brother. He was twenty years old at the time. Since he was older, I also started picking up the habits that he had. I started drinking heavily because everybody else around me was drinking. Drowning my insides with alcohol helped stop the pain I was feeling inside of myself. It numbed things, and made it so that I could only think about anything other than what had happened to me and the direction my life was going in.

I thought alcohol was the answer to all my problems. By the time I was eighteen years old, I was an alcoholic; I was drinking top shelf, hard liquor on a regular basis. I drank EVERYTHING!!! My friend's brother and I drank together a lot; he was my man, and I was mimicking his behavior. We both were addicted to liquor, and soon he became a mean drunk. When he was in *that* mood, it did not take much for me to set him off. It was not long into the relationship before he started hitting me and giving me black eyes.

What could I do? I didn't have anyone and I didn't have anywhere to go, so I stayed.

Drinking became an everyday habit for me. It was the only way I knew how to cope. I started working by going to the fields to pick tomatoes and peppers. It was the only way I knew how to legally make money. Working in the fields didn't pay much though. I only made enough money to keep myself supplied with something to drink daily; there wasn't much left for anything else.

One day, the brother of the man that I was going out with, hit me in the face and broke my nose. I still stayed. Staying in abusive relationships was becoming my norm. Fear had taken over my whole being, and no one was helping me overcome it. I didn't know what to do. My soul was crying, and I was drinking more and more – self-medicating myself in order to cope.

Don't copy the behavior and customs of this world, but let God transform you into a new person by changing the way you think. Then you will be able to discern what is good, pleasing, and the perfect will of God. Romans 12:2

In my twenties, I had lost all touch with reality. I couldn't think straight. I couldn't see. I hurt all over and I needed to stop the pain. The money I was making from picking peppers was not enough, and I was tired of working really hard for chump change. I took the focus of my pain and put it on my body. I was pretty, with a cute face and a slamming body. I was literally sitting on a moneymaker, so I slept with men for money. A lot of men were interested in me, but I wasn't interested in them. The only thing that I cared about was the money I could get from them for my next drink. I hated when I had to sleep with those men, but I had to do what I had to do in order to survive. Most of the men were married, but they treated me with kindness and what I thought, at the time, was love. I never thought I was doing anything wrong. I was just trying to find someone to take care of that lost little girl inside of me. I was exchanging what they desired – my body – for what I thought was financial support and love. It seemed like a fair trade. Only problem was that I was not receiving love from them. They were buying property; or at least leasing it, and sometimes they felt that they could do anything they felt like doing with the property they purchased. I was even hit once or twice by some of the married men. I saw myself, at that time, as a crazy person; someone just existing, but not living…so none of it mattered. I had no one who cared, and no one to tell my story to anyway.

So I am not the one doing wrong, it is sin living in me that does it. And I know that nothing good lives in me, this is my sinful nature. I want to do what is right, but I can't. I want do what is good, but I don't. I don't want to do what is wrong, but I do it anyway. Romans 7:17-19

*****

Never enough

Somehow, I ended up living back with my family after many years. I was broke and could not be fixed. I pretended to be happy; but how could that be, when I never experienced that type of union with anyone; blood or otherwise? I would be in a room full of family members and would feel so lonely. Sometimes, I would leave just to go somewhere to cry.

Why didn't anybody love me?

I felt anger and rage building up inside of me, and no one could see how unhappy I truly was.

Why could no one see my pain?
Why didn't anyone know I was so lost, lonely, and afraid?
Why didn't anyone care?
Why didn't anyone rescue me?

There were no answers, but the mask I wore seemed to allow me to be accepted, so I became this perfect little girl just so I could feel some resemblance of belonging. I made sure that everything about me on the outside was just right. I wore my mask for a long time.

I lived with my cousin, Andrea – the sister of the man who raped me. By that time, I had moved back with my family, and I had suppressed the rape incident so far back in my mind that I stopped thinking about it. The alcohol took care of those thoughts.

In 1991, my cousin kicked me out of her house. She said she did it because I didn't want to work and babysit her children or grandchildren. The truth of the matter was, on that particular day, I was sent home from work because I was sick. The children she wanted me to babysit were not her grandchildren. They had someone to watch them. It was not my duty to take care of them, but she used that as an excuse for something else that was going on. She wanted me gone. They all did; and it was only a matter of time before they made that happen. I was unwanted and I knew that I would always have to stand on my own; I had no real family to help me or encourage me, and the people in the home where I was living were tired of acting like they cared about me. When I got into an argument with one family member, the whole family would gang up on me. It was *them* against *me*. I was an outsider, and that hurt.

I tell you the truth, you will weep and mourn over what is going to happen to me, but the world will rejoice. I will grieve, but my grief will suddenly turn to wonderful joy. John 16:20

So, there I was, back on the streets in the middle of winter, and in the middle of the night. I ended up living with a young woman who was a drug addict. A week after I moved in with her, I came home from work and she wasn't there. I sat down to eat my lunch, and this great pain hit me all of a sudden in my abdomen. I was on the floor for about ten minutes before she came home. I was rushed to the hospital and had emergency surgery. Come to find out, my appendix had burst. I believe if she had not come home at the time that she did, I would have died. I stayed in the hospital for two months. The doctors said I needed someone to take care of me. I told my cousin, the same one who had kicked me out, what the doctor said.

She said to me, "Did you tell them that you don't have anyone to take care of you?" There was no sympathy or concern in her voice.

Instantly, my heart broke into two pieces after hearing what I had already known to be true concerning my family. They didn't give a damn about me, and they didn't care if I knew it.

I ended up staying with a man named Haywood. He was an older man and a good friend; the father figure that I always wanted. He saw how lonely I was, and he knew I was hurt by my cousin's words. Once he even told me that he could see that nobody in my life had ever taken the time to teach me anything about life. He was right! That is why I was so mixed up in the head.

Haywood tried to teach me how to handle money and men. He would say things to me like, "If a man can't buy you a bedroom set, the hell with him." The truth of the matter is, I never had to ask for anything from men, they always seemed to buy me everything I wanted. I didn't know that their gifts were bait to keep me to themselves. I was naive and believed that their gifts meant they cared. Reality is, they were using me just as much as I was using them.

Haywood died a few years before I got arrested for the crime that I am now incarcerated for. He tried to help me. He was probably the only person on this Earth who tried to help me out until I took up residence within these four walls. He tried…but I think our paths crossed too late in my life for it to make a significant difference. I will always miss him. When he died, I remember feeling that I didn't want to be here anymore on this Earth.

God…I was so lonely.

*****

Actions Collide

From the point of my childhood molestation on, I just seemed to attract partners who constantly abused me physically, as well as mentally. When I lived in South Jersey, my boyfriend at that time beat me. My siblings never witnessed any of his assaults on me, but I was seen sporting two black eyes during that time, and I am sure they could surmise where those black eyes came from. Another one of the men I was involved with struck me over the head with a trashcan, causing another serious injury to my head. Yet another male friend slit my face with a knife.

Abuse on top of abuse, on top of abuse. That was my life.

It's no wonder why I drank so much.

That is why we never give up. Though our bodies are dying, our spirits are being renewed every day. For our present troubles are small and won't last very long. 2 Corinthians 4:16-17

70

I didn't understand why I was suffering so much; but through it all, God intervened to save me. Then I was hit in the head with a trashcan, my shoulder bone broke and shortly after that, I was cut in the face with a butcher knife. Even as a little girl, I was hit in the head with something sharp.

The only question I ever wanted to know the answer to was…*why did I have to endure so much pain and suffering?*

I must admit, I have always felt the presence of something or someone around me. I was so messed up that I didn't pay attention to whatever it was. I just kept living in a dark world.

You will grope around in broad daylight like a blind person groping in the darkness, but you will not find your way. You will be oppressed and robbed continually and no one will come to save you. Deuteronomy 28:29

I am here, behind these prison walls, because something terrible was happening to me yet again. Another rape. *The same crime perpetrated on the same person three times…it has to be me…that's* what I told myself as it happened…AGAIN. A mind can only take so much torment. Memories of pain can only be buried so deep before they rise to the surface. Even a loyal dog will only take so much abuse before it bites back at its master. Unfortunately, I became that dog.

In the midst of being a victim once again, the pain became too much to bear. I couldn't silence the pain or bury it again. As I felt my soul being raped again and used at will, the little girl inside me cried, *NO MORE!!!*

God responded in unison with me, "No more."

A life was lost and someone else lived. At that moment, I wanted to be saved from the abuse, from the misery, and from the pain; but not at the extent of accidentally taking someone's life. Having done so is a horrible feeling to live with. I still don't know how to feel about that; I guess I'll never feel right.

*****

The Day That Changed Things Forever

I met Ernest one day while over at my cousin's house. He kept making passes at me and would sometimes box me in a corner so I would notice him. I lived a couple of doors away from my cousin, but I didn't come to her house much because, just like when I was around the rest of my family, when I was around her I felt unwanted and unloved most of the time, so I tried to save myself from more misery. Even though I didn't go over my cousin's house a lot, that didn't stop Ernest from making more moves on me.

One day, Ernest came to my apartment unannounced; he had a thirty-pack of beer and a fifth of liquor. I hadn't given him much attention before that, but that didn't seem to matter, Ernest made it a point of initiating a relationship between us.

That was the beginning for us. It was a done deal when he showed up at my door with liquor because he had managed to give my weak spot what it needed. He had liquor…and I was an alcoholic. It was as simple as that. That's all that was needed to win me over. I was very vulnerable at the time, and blind to deception. I must say that when I looked at Ernest as he walked up that day with the beer and liquor in his hand, I felt that something just was not right about him. My spirit told me as much, but I dismissed my feelings as I always did. We drank, danced, laughed, and had sex that day. I liked Ernest. He made me laugh and we liked the same foods. It seemed like we had a lot in common; most notably, the fact that he was an addict and I was an alcoholic – an alcoholic with very low self-esteem.

I craved for someone to love me, and the first three months with Ernest were okay because he showed me the love that I thought I needed. My apartment was like a party place. Different people were there every day drinking and smoking weed; but even with all that was going on at my place, Ernest hid his serious drug use from me.

It wasn't long after that when the sexual abuse started. It started passive at first. I would be asleep on the couch sometimes and all of a sudden, Ernest would be standing over top of me naked, and he would make me have sex. He would say that I was supposed to have sex with him because I was *his* woman. He seemed to think that he owned me, and that my body was his to do what he pleased.

After sex was over, I would feel some type of way toward him forcing himself on me, but I didn't know how to stop it. Sometimes when he took sex from me without my consent, I would put him out of my place, but he would always come back apologizing, and I would let him back in. Most of the time after those incidents occurred, Ernest would sweet talk me, buy me plants, flowers, and other gifts to apologize and show me that he cared, and after that, things would be okay between us again for a while. Then the physical fighting would start all over again. He would hit me, and sometimes I would hit him back. Sometimes I won, and many times I lost. In between the physical fighting and arguing, the relationship became worst; it was really bad.

Time went on, we continued to argue, and even the lady that lived upstairs started stomping on the floor to tell us to shut up. I got frustrated and told Ernest to get out of my apartment. He kept saying things about my old boyfriend still being in my life, and that my old boyfriend was causing trouble in our relationship.

Things got really bad the day that changed my life forever. Ernest and I were hollering, screaming, yelling, and drinking. I went outside to get some air, and a neighbor pulled up; she was coming home from work. We talked a little bit and eventually went to the liquor store. When we came back, we went into my apartment, sat down, and began drinking and talking some more. Ernest came from the back room talking crazy, and he and I started arguing again.

The neighbor stayed for another ten minutes or so, then she said, "I'm leaving. I don't want to hear all that noise."

I was angry that she was leaving, and I got up and went straight into the kitchen to finish cooking. After a few minutes, Ernest came out of the back room and he was naked from the waist down.

He said, "I want to be with my lady."

From the day we were already having, I knew that I did not want to have sex with him. I said, "Later. We have all night."

Ernest didn't want to hear that. The more I said, "Wait," the more enraged he became. I started getting irritated and frustrated and out of anger I said, "The hell with it." I came out of the kitchen angry and said, "Fuck it" and I laid down on the couch mad and fully dressed. I was going to let him rape me. Anything to make the arguing stop.

Ernest took advantage of the situation and got on top of me talking crazy and manhandling me. After it was over, I started to wrestle him off of me. What happened after that is kind of a blur. I'm not sure, but I think he fell on the floor and I ran to the back of my bedroom. I locked the door behind me. I was scared.

I sat on the bed saying, "God, why is he doing this?"

Things got loud in the living room and I heard Ernest turn up the music. I unlocked the door quietly, and slowly walked down the hallway. I didn't see Ernest when I got to the entrance of the living room, so I grabbed my coat from the couch, unlocked the front door, and ran out the door headed to the stairs of the apartment building. As I approached the second set of stairs, Ernest came out of nowhere. Before I knew it, he was pulling me back down the steps, trying to get me back into my apartment. We wrestled down the steps. He got me back inside my apartment, and we continued fighting in the front doorway.

I was trying to get back to my bedroom and Ernest was trying to stop me. We continued fighting all the way down the hallway, and he pushed me up against the wall in front of the bathroom. Then he began choking me. As I was gasping for air, I remembered that I had an old fashion can opener on my key chain. I pulled it out, and cut Ernest down his neck with it. I don't know how bad the cut was, but it was long.

Ernest let me go. He went into the bathroom and I went and locked myself in the bedroom. At first, I sat on the bed shaking...scared and nervous. Then I got up and tried to climb out the window. The blinds fell down, which stopped me because of the noise it was making. Ernest was outside the bedroom screaming that he should kick the bathroom door down, and telling me that I better not climb out the window. A few minutes later, I heard the front door open and close.

I unlocked the bedroom door and started walking down the hallway saying, "Thank you, God...he's gone."

Thinking he was out of the apartment, I calmed down a bit. I went to the stove and turned it on; deciding to finish dinner. Before I knew what was happening, Ernest came from around the corner and cornered me in the kitchen.

He turned the stove off and said, "Now you're going to give me some of this pussy." He was grabbing at my T-shirt while looking at me with devilish, threatening eyes.

I don't remember picking up the knife from the stove. All I remember is that he was pulling me down the hall saying, "You're going to give me some."

I looked down and saw the knife being held tightly in my hand. I couldn't drop it. Something inside me made me hold on to it tighter.

I pulled back from Ernest as best I could, but he got me down the hall, into the bedroom, and he pushed me onto the bed. He took off my shoes and started taking my clothes off. I was frozen. My body betrayed me and would not move. I sat on the bed with the knife under my thigh. I was hiding it from Ernest as he ripped my clothes off. My panties, my long johns, my sweat pants...they were all being pulled off of me at the same time. He moved like a mad man on a mission. His actions were in a frenzy.

Ernest pushed me back on the bed and was mounting himself on top of me. Everything was in slow motion, and I started kicking him. He took and put his knee on my chest to hold me down; forcing me to be still.

I started hollering, "Help...help me!"

No one heard me, but I continued to scream nonetheless.

Ernest put his hand over my mouth and told me to shut up. I was hollering for the neighbor upstairs to call the police. Ernest continued coming down on me, and I started kicking, swinging my arms wildly, and trying my best to fight him off of me.

We were enemies at war; both determined to win.

The next thing I remember is Ernest saying, "Uh...now," and he punched me in the stomach and climbed off of me. We both doubled over in pain.

I took in several deep breaths from his blow, trying to quench the pain. When my stomach stopped hurting, I jumped up, grabbed another pair of pants, rushed putting them on, and I ran down the hall and out the door...hollering and screaming all the way.

*****

On July 2, 2004, my life changed forever as a judge hit a gavel on his bench, sentencing me to sixty years in prison for Ernest's death. I have been locked up for fourteen years now, and I can only keep hoping and praying that one day I will receive JUSTICE. But while

I am waiting, I will do my best to remain faithful to God and to keep looking for something good in all of this.

*****

Feelings in the Aftermath

I've been asked often how did I feel after the incident.

Was I dazed?
Numb?
What went across my mind?
Was I afraid?

To be honest, I don't remember feeling anything. I was empty, and I immediately began to drift away. At that moment, while I was bent over and leaning on the fence outside of my apartment waiting for the police to come…people were everywhere, but no one heard me hollering and screaming for help.

One of the witnesses came out of my apartment and said, "Don't run now." The voice was accusing and judgmental.

Little did the witness know…I was not going anywhere. I couldn't move; nor did I feel a need to do so. I was an observer to what had happened just like everyone else was. I only moved when the police came and took me back into the apartment. I willingly went with them. I did not fear them, or what was inside the apartment. I could not comprehend what had happened, or that it had happened because of my actions. I couldn't hear as they asked me questions. I saw their lips moving, but I did not understand what they were saying. I guess I can describe it as…I was there, yet not there at the same time. I knew something ugly had happened, but I had no guilt about what happened or why.

All I know is that at that moment, as the police were questioning me, I felt that same way I did long before…the same way I felt when my cousin raped me in my sleep over thirty-five years earlier. Paralyzed was more like how I felt; like I was falling.

By the time I was taken to the police station and the questions continued, all I remember is giving yes and no answers. Those answers didn't come from a place of being rebellious, smug, or even trying to protect myself from incriminating myself. I gave the police the only answers I was capable of giving. I tried to tell them what happened, but I couldn't remember the details. To be honest, I couldn't remember most of the incident at all. I was drifting away; distancing myself from the moment that the pain became too hard to bear and protection mode took control. I was as honest with them as my observer point of view would allow me to be.

When the police informed me that Ernest didn't "make it," all I could do was drift further away. I wasn't afraid because my mind was empty. I didn't say anything...I just sat there empty.

*****

I've Been Changed

How am I a changed person?

When living outside of incarcerated walls, I was in the midst of my own personal hell. I struggled each day in trying to figure out who I was. Where I belonged was an everyday challenge that I tried desperately to conquer. I was searching for answers that never came. I realize now that I come from a dysfunctional family. I am in no position to blame my family for my hurts, habits, and hang-ups. It's hard to accept, but I do. I love my family. I am free from my past. These are not just words. I am a new person.

When I think about the old Marvella, I shake my head; not in shame, but in this new hope that I have for myself. You may believe me or not, but this discipline I now experience, I accept with open arms. I am convinced that it comes from above. I have learned that I am stronger than I ever gave myself credit for. I am in charge of my life, even behind prison walls. I don't rely on my own understanding. I have a good relationship with Jesus. I am changed; I am free; and I have been given a second chance to live right, love right, and forgive right.

Don't get me wrong...I'll always carry remorse for Ernest and the loss of his life. I continually pray for his soul. I try every day to be aware of the evils of the world so that I will never harm anyone again; not even myself. I have learned that I have many gifts and talents, and that they were hidden for many, many, years. That's what living in darkness does to you. It makes you blind to reality, and the world around you. But thank God for His grace and mercy; because the evil one did not want me to live. But I survived, and I will keep on surviving; yes, even in here.

Anyone who assaults and kills another person must be put to death. But if it was simply an accident permitted by God, I will appoint a place of refuge where the slayer can run for safety. Exodus 21:12-13

When I turned my life over to Jesus Christ, I realized that through all the pain, suffering, loneliness, sadness, and abandonment...He was with me all the time.

For a brief moment, I abandoned you, but with great compassion I will take you back. In a burst of anger, I turned my face away for a little while. But with everlasting love, I will have compassion on you says the Lord, your redeemer. Isiah 54:7-8

Since I have been in recovery, the things that used to bother and worry me are like dust. I was a stranger to my family for a few years. I blamed my family for most of the things that happened to me in my life, and I wanted someone to hurt in the same manner in which I was hurting. Then I remembered...*judge not, lest ye be judged*. I recognize now that they were suffering and struggling with their own addictions; they were in no place to help me, because they were trying to help themselves.

Recovery helped me see that.

O Merciful One, I place my hands into you so that together we can do something that I cannot do alone. God, grant me the serenity to accept the things I cannot change, the courage to change the things I can, and the wisdom to know the difference. Amen.

As I sit in a place that is known for stunting a person's ability to grow and succeed, I am enjoying how God is helping me make positive changes in my life. On the outside, I didn't realize how important it was to keep going in my recovery groups; but now I understand how a recovery group helps me look at the past and learn how to grow from it while making decisions in my life.

Before being here, I didn't want to accept change; I didn't want to grow. All I wanted was for someone to understand and feel the suffering and pain I had endured. I wanted to stay in my past; in the deep dark place that I had begun to call home. To tell you the truth, before I started recovery in here, I got along just fine with the rest of the women in here. I think that was because I was okay wallowing in self-pity and misery. I didn't care anything about growing. All I cared about was making someone understand my pain. That feeling was universal with most of the women here, so we got along fine. But now, I am lucky if I get a decent conversation. Some of the women don't understand my change. They say I don't act right, or that I have changed too much because I don't hang around the same crowd that I used to. I walk away smiling; letting them know that the person they are looking for is gone. That was the old me. The only attention I need now is Jesus Christ.

Of course, your former friends are surprised when you no longer plunge into the flood of wild and destructive things they do. So they slander you. 1 Peter 4:4

To this day, I still think about and remember that horrible night in 2001. I was so broken hearted about what happened, that I don't think I truly understood what occurred. All I thought about was the fact that God was going to forgive me. I cried so much that they put me on medication. I felt like nothing. I didn't even think I did anything wrong because I kept asking if I could I go home.

I was so empty; I had nothing, not even myself. But even in the midst of all that, I felt love from above and I knew that God would forgive His child. He knows my heart. He knows my fears. He knows my transgressions. He knows my pain.

So, yes…I have forgiven myself, because I know Jesus has forgiven me.

Fear not; you will no longer live in shame. Don't be afraid, there is no more disgrace for you. Isaiah 54:4 Read forgiveness Psalm 103; 1-22

When I started attending recovery, I was at my lowest point in life, and I needed to gain my sanity back. I've been convicted of the most heinous of crimes, and I needed forgiveness. Recovery has helped me realize that I am not a bad person. I am just a person that bad things have happened to. But in that realization, I also have to accept that everyone has to take responsibility for their actions.

I was weak in a lot of areas of my life. I believed my weakest point was in not being able to forgive my family for protecting my cousin when he raped me. I realized, through my recovery process, that I have a story to tell. I realized that all the abuse I've endured as a child, teenager, and an adult, will not go in vain. I realized that suffering in silence is not the answer.

And since, I, the Lord and teacher, have washed your feet, you ought to wash each other's feet. I have given you an example to follow, do as I have done to you. John 13:14-15

As much as I put blame on my family and my upbringing for the evils that have occurred in my life, I also realize that I need them in my life in order to heal and grow; and that God is slowly working that out for the good in my life.

Then Esau ran to meet him (Jacob) and embraced him, threw his arms around his neck and kissed him, and they both wept. Genesis 33:4

Chapter Three

Dominique's Story:
Sexual Abuse from A Different Perspective

The most common question that's always asked is, "Why...why did they do it?"

History has a way of repeating itself; the good, bad and the ugly. This chapter, will hopefully shed some light on what happens when child sexual abuse goes untreated. Not every victim will go on to be abusers; however, there are some that will repeat the cycle. Dominique's story may help us to better understand what goes on in the mind of an abuser, and what leads some to selfishly violate others.

I had mixed feelings about the idea of interviewing a convicted sex offender because I didn't know what emotions I would experience by confronting someone who committed the same crime that caused me so much pain and suffering.

However, I could not let fear stop me from accomplishing the mission I was supposed to fulfill. That meant stepping into territory I was uncomfortable crossing into. It was necessary to hear about sexual abuse from the other side—from someone who had been a perpetrator in causing abuse. This information would shed some light, and maybe even answer some questions for me and others in understanding why, and what goes on in a perpetrator's mind.

I also realized that this interview might well provide an opportunity for a breakthrough in my own personal healing process, and to educate me in the field that I am pursuing.

The interview below took place at the Adult Diagnostic Treatment Center (ADTC) in Avenel, New Jersey; a prison that houses and provides treatment for approximately 767 male sex offenders. Dominique is a thirty-three-year-old Hispanic/African-American male who volunteered to tell his story. His name has been changed to protect his identity.

*****

When I first met Dominique, I found him to be articulate and polite—just a regular guy. He had received a twenty-year sentence for sexually abusing his sister and his son. He had already served ten years of that sentence when I met him; eight of which were spent at ADTC.

He said he wanted to be included in my project in order to put out some positive energy to help people who suffer from the effects of having been sexually abused.

Dominique was one of three children; with one older brother, and a younger sister who was almost a decade younger than him, he always believed his father showed favoritism toward his sister, which made him resentful and angry.

Dominique began talking to me with an explanation of why he had agreed to be interviewed.

"My life has taught me a lot. When I think about all the energy I spent on the street, doing things I shouldn't have been doing, I decided to try to turn it around by putting out some positive energy that might help me and others."

I thanked him again for agreeing to do the interview and went on to explain that I believed a sex offender's view of sexual abuse would help give my book some balance. I asked him if there had been any sexual trauma in his life – a common factor, which motivates many sexual offenders. He told me yes; he had experienced sexual trauma as a young boy. He began his story by telling me more about his childhood, and the first time his cousin sexually abused him.

"I was born in Italy. My family was in the military, so we moved around a lot. We lived abroad until we moved to New Jersey in 1979, where we lived on base. Then we moved back to Europe in 1986 and stayed there another three years. We moved back to New Jersey in 1990, and I've been here ever since.

"My father retired from the military and is now a church pastor. My mother is a schoolteacher. I am their middle child, with an older brother and a younger sister.

"Looking back, I would say I grew up in an ideal, almost perfect family. We ate our meals together, took family vacations, and even had family meetings every Friday. I had a happy childhood until the day I found out my father had cheated on my mother – something that sent a huge negative ripple through all of our lives.

"It was then that we went down to visit my aunt, uncle, and cousins in Baltimore one weekend; something we had done before. Whenever we went down there, we'd always take showers on Saturday night to get ready for church on Sunday morning.

"That weekend, when my cousin, who was nine at the time, suggested we shower together, I agreed to do so. I continued to agree when he suggested we practice, in the shower, some of the wrestling moves we had seen on TV. It was at that point that he started touching me between my legs, and then put me on top of him, where he began to tickle and fondle me.

"I wasn't sure what was going on; many different feelings ran through my head when my aunt called us to get out of the shower. We went to his room to get dressed, but my cousin wanted to keep on wrestling. I agreed, but I never expected to end up on his bed, where he made me give him oral sex.

"Sex in general was very secretive back then. But as exciting as it was, this kind of sex did not feel good to me. When I told him I wanted to stop, he agreed. Then we both went to sleep. The next day after church, in my grandfather's house, my cousin tried to rape me. I was in the bedroom taking off my Sunday clothes when he came from behind and bent me over the bed, pulled my underwear down, and then got ready to penetrate me. Fortunately, my grandfather came up, and asked what we were doing. I was trembling, but my cousin was cool and collected.

"Just playing around," he told my grandfather, who believed him and went out of the room.

"Later, as we were going downstairs, my cousin leaned over and whispered in my ear, "Gotcha'!

"It was at that point that I got scared. I tried to stay around the rest of the family for the rest of the weekend so I didn't have to be alone with my cousin.

"He somehow managed to get me alone later that day. We were downstairs playing *Twister* when he asked me to put my hands on him. I didn't want to do it, but I didn't want to challenge him either. He was older than I was…and bigger too. I couldn't help but feel a little bit afraid of him. I ended up giving him more oral sex that day. I had put my clothes back on by the time my brother came downstairs, so he never realized what had happened."

Dominique went on to say how his mother spoke to him about sex three years later; right before the family was scheduled to move back to Europe.

"I was almost ten years old when my mother said, 'Let's go down to the library and get some books on sex education.'

"After we went to the library, she asked if I had any questions. That was when I remembered what my cousin had done to me. 'What if someone puts their hands on you and you don't like it?' I asked her.

"My mother just shook her head. 'Dominique,' she said, '…there's always something going on with you. It's always about you. What about me…and the fact that your father cheated on me?' she asked before she burst into tears.

"Bad news! If I had any hope of telling her how my cousin had abused me, it went right out the door and I knew then it wasn't going to happen. Meanwhile, my mother was still crying. I did my best to console her. I gave her a hug; privately, I also made up in my mind that there was no sense telling anyone what had happened to me or how it made me feel."

I asked Dominique if the abuse had continued in those three years between the time it first happened and when the family's moved back to Europe.

He replied, "No. It only happened those two times that one week-end. Thankfully, after that, we stopped going to Baltimore."

Dominique, as if in a trance, went on to tell me more about his family's move to Europe.

"We moved to Europe then—away from all my friends. But my brother and I still felt the move was a good thing; there was so much chaos in our family back then, that we felt the move would give us all a new beginning. My brother and I really hoped things would get better.

"Our first six months abroad were wonderful. My father would take us to breakfast every Saturday morning, and me and my mother actually began to get along pretty well. Everything was going fine until my father received some notoriety from him being a minister while serving in the military. At that point, we were back to square one. The family no longer ate together as much; there was less communication. It was around that time that my sister was born; adding a whole new set of problems to our lives."

Dominique went on to describe one example of those problems.

"I remember one time when I had football practice. We lived in a German neighborhood about twenty minutes away from the American neighborhood. It took a good thirty minutes to get to football practice.

"One night after practice, the coach offered to drive me home when no one came to pick me up. I assured him my mother would be there, but practice ended at seven o'clock and she didn't show up until eight thirty. It was raining that night; I was crying by the time she got there.

"'I'm sorry, Dominique, I forgot about you,' she said. Those words hurt me deeply. I felt like nobody cared. I went to my room as soon as we got home. I felt like no one could hurt me there; it was my own personal, protective cocoon.

"It was at that point that I began to question if my new baby sister was, in fact, really my sister. My father had spoken to me before she was born, telling me, 'Listen, this is your sister. So whatever you're thinking, you can't do it.'

"I still don't know exactly what he was thinking, or how he even came up with feeling the need to say what he said to me, but I do remember the way he was always protecting her.

"'Oh, that's a princess, there! Nobody's going to lay a hand on my Princess,' he'd say over and over again after she was born. Each time he said it, it made me feel angry, resentful, and disconnected. Very simply put, I felt as if I had lost my father, the parent I was closest to, since I had never gotten along that well with my mother.

"Nor did my mother and father get along at that time. If my father told me to come home at 8:00 p.m., for example, my mother might say, 'Come home at 8:30 p.m.' They were always giving me those kinds of mixed messages.

"That was why after my sister was born, and was clearly favored by my father, I started to believe I might not be my parents' natural child; instead, I believed I was adopted. That was why whenever my parents went out, I'd go through their drawers trying to find proof of my adoption. Because if I really had been adopted, at least that would explain what was going on, and why I felt so disconnected, as if I was the black sheep of the family."

Dominique went on to explain how his racial heritage and skin color reinforced those feelings within him.

"My family was mixed. My mother was African-American and my father was a dark-skinned Hispanic. In terms of color, my mother was lighter than me, and my brother was also light-skinned with green eyes. I was definitely the darkest-skinned person in the family, which was the main reason I believed I really might have been adopted."

Dominique never found any evidence which indicated he actually was adopted; but after his sister was born and favored by his father, his growing resentment resulted in more problems.

"I was nine when my sister was born. I soon began to resent my father. With my new baby sister getting all his attention, I felt unloved, ignored, and neglected. I began to ask myself how I could regain my father's attention and love. That was when I started looking at my sister in a sexual way.

"The house was set up so that you had to go through my sister's room to get to my parents' room and my room too. Meanwhile, I had begun to drink alcohol. That happened when my parents' landlord asked me to take care of the horses he kept in back of the house. He would reward me by letting me ride them, and also giving me a key to his liquor cabinet. The rules about sex, drugs, and alcohol were a lot more lenient in Europe than they were in the United States; so, drinking at that age was not frowned upon.

"In any case, whenever my parents kept me up at night with their arguments, I would escape to my landlord's place—and his liquor. But really, being by myself at those times, was just as important to me as drinking the liquor.

"This went on for a couple of years. I was eleven when I noticed his VCR player and a shelf with some videotapes on it. I put one of the tapes in that night. It was a porno tape. I was soon watching the tapes often, and no one knew I was doing it. I never expected how quickly the tapes would trigger sexual feelings in me; and yet, at the same time, they triggered shame for having those sexual feelings."

Dominique said that those feelings eventually caused him to begin to abuse his little sister, and he explained how that came about.

"One night after I had a few drinks and watched a porno video at my landlord's house, I went through my sister's room to get to my own room. I saw her lying in bed; she was three years old at that time.

"It was a hot night and I remember looking at her, sexually, for the first time. Those sexual thoughts did not make me happy, and I tried to repress them. I told myself to keep right on going past her room. But that night, when I got to my room, I masturbated to the fantasy of molesting my sister.

"The next morning, my mother had a huge argument with my father and slapped him so hard it left marks on his face and he left. That made me so angry and something deep inside me snapped.

"I went into my sister's room and asked her if she wanted to come into my room to play a video game. She said, "okay." She was wearing a long t-shirt that day. I used the same tactics with her that my cousin had used with me. Looking back…it embarrasses me to say it, but I laid her down on her stomach and said, 'C'mon, let's wrestle.' Then I took her shirt off and pulled her panties down. I then took out my penis and moved back and forth between the cheeks of her backside until I came. Then I got up and pretended everything was okay.

"She left without another word and the rest of that day went on as if nothing unusual had happened. I never planned to do it again, but a few weeks later, that's exactly what happened. But this time, it was late afternoon, and my father came home unexpectedly and caught me molesting my sister.

"'What are you doing? What's going on?' he demanded. The answer was simple; he and I both knew what I was doing. I remember screaming out, 'This is wrong. I need help!'

"I never expected my father's reply. 'No, it's just your hormones. You're eleven years old, in a new country—experiencing different things.' I guessed that meant he was okay with what I had done, which was important to me because my father's word was law back then. There never was any punishment or repercussion for what I had done. I was still nervous about what might happen if I ever did it again…that was the reason why I never did again; at least not while we were still living in Europe."

Dominique's family returned to New Jersey three years later, when he was fourteen and his sister was five or six. He talked about the family's return and the return of his abuse of his sister.

"The night after we moved back, my mother and father had to go to a military ball. My father asked me to watch my sister, and I agreed, even though in the back of my mind, I knew I should not be alone with her. Since it was my father who had asked, I thought it must be okay. However, that turned out not to be the case. The same thing happened that night that had happened in Europe. I brought her up to my bedroom and molested her.

"I asked her if she was frightened. She wasn't scared because I made it feel like a game – the 'under the covers game;' that's what I called it. So as soon as I suggested we play, she agreed. I hate to say it, but I guess I had trained her, bringing her to the point where it all seemed normal. Meanwhile, deep inside, I told myself that even though my father might think of her as his Princess, really, she was as low as I was because she never put up a fight and never resisted me in any way.

"I wrestled with that issue, but not for long. Everything felt all right until my parents came home. My sister was in the bathroom when they noticed her underwear were on inside out.

"'Did you do it again?' my father asked. When I said 'yes,' he replied that he thought he should send me to a detention center for boys.

"'Hold on. Three years ago it wasn't an issue, and now, all of a sudden, it is?' I replied. Looking back, I know how manipulative that was. I knew I was essentially blackmailing my father in terms of affecting his strong, very positive public image. At that time, my father was really tight with the general who lived on the Army base. So when he threatened to send me away, I knew he would have to ask the General for permission; something he would never, ever, do because that would reveal our family's problems.

"That was why he walked out of my room, slamming the door behind him. After that, we didn't speak to each other for the next week."

I asked Dominique where his brother was at the time all of this was going on, and how he was involved in the situation.

"My brother knew what was going on; everyone did. They swept it under the rug; it was a huge family secret. Nobody talked about it because the last thing my parents wanted was for that kind of truth to ever get out. That was the way my father was raised—never air dirty family laundry.

"Another strange thing was that my parents were very strict with us as we were growing up. All of our lives, everyone we knew, and everything we did, had to be connected with the church—that was a very strong foundation for my family. My father was also such a reg-imented person – probably from being in the military – so he insisted that we keep to a firm schedule even in the summer. I remember several years when we had vacation Bible school from 9:00 a.m. to 11:00 a.m., homework from 12:00 p.m. to 4:00 p.m., and more Bible school from 6:00 p.m. to 8:00 p.m. at night.

"My father directed our church attendance on Sundays just as rigidly. We couldn't sit in the pews with our friends; we had to sit with the family. If there was anything scheduled after church, we had to go to that too. At some point, I felt lonely; then I got angry over it. I felt very isolated at this point. My father always told us we couldn't trust anyone outside the family. Since I wasn't getting along with anyone in my family, at that time, I just began to spend a lot of time in my room; the room I had started to think of as my sanctuary."

Dominique went on to explain how that feeling of isolation had begun after his cousin molested him, which was also right around the same time his father cheated on his mother.

"Everything went downhill after my cousin raped me. We were a happy family before that happened; my parents would always say how lucky they were to have children like us. Then, my father cheated on my mother with the choir director. Both events caused all kinds of problems among us, and I felt like we were five strangers living in the same house.

"It got so bad that sometimes, my mother would pack us up in the car and drive around New Jersey looking for a new church to attend. We were Baptist, so those were the churches we went to. No matter where we went, we soon found that they knew who my father was and they had respect for him."

Dominique went back to talking about the way he molested his sister. I asked how he felt about what he had done as he looked back on it. Then we went on to the subject of forgiveness.

"Looking back on that part of my life, I am extremely embarrassed. I also feel lots of guilt and remorse because I took out my painful feelings on an innocent person; someone who did not deserve it; someone who didn't even know what was going on.

"I felt blessed, four or five years ago, when they had a Family Day here, and my mother and my sister – who was eighteen at that time – came up. When my mother went to use the bathroom, my sister told me she forgave me.

"*You shouldn't be saying that*, I wanted to tell her. *You should be cursing me out.*

"It really wasn't about her. The problem was I had never forgiven myself for what I had done. I'm very thankful today that my sister and I have a solid relationship. I still have lots of regret and guilt; I know I never should have done it."

At that point, I asked Dominique if he felt he would ever be able to forgive himself for what he had done.

"I'm in that stage now, and I'm trying my best. I'm not all the way there…not yet."

I went on to ask him if he felt he could ever forgive his cousin.

"That's still a sore spot, but I know that if I were to see him again, I could never refuse to speak to him. It would also be tough to stay mad at him when my own sister has forgiven me. That would be selfish on my part.

"*If she can forgive me, why can't I forgive him?* I ask myself that question often—that's how I'm working on forgiving him. I want to let it go, whether I ever see him again or not. I want to be in that place of forgiveness."

Dominique went on to tell me more about his relationships with others, including the mother of his children.

"I was sixteen when I met this girl and we began to have a relationship outside the church. She and I were very involved with each other for the next six years. When I was seventeen and she was nineteen, we had our first child out of wedlock. Of course, my father didn't like that. I didn't like the way he acted when he first found out she was pregnant. After spending so much of his life preaching against abortion, I was stunned when he told me privately, one day, that he thought this woman should go out and do just that—abort our child.

"That baby, a son, turned out to be the first of our two children. Our relationship was never easy. She and I ran away right before our first baby was born because neither of our families could accept our relationship. Our family was upscale and prestigious. Everyone knew and respected my father. My girlfriend came from a very different kind of family, with a mother who was always in and out of jail. Part of the reason I loved her had to do with the fact that she was definitely someone I could rescue. I loved the way she looked up to me and my family because of who we were and how much we had. Very few people had ever looked up to me before—for any reason.

"After we ran away, and before our son was born, we lived with a friend. It was at that time that my father got me a job working in a warehouse making pretty good money; enough to enable us to move out and finally get our own place. I remember one night, I brought my son over to my family's house. My mother looked at us and said, 'I'm going to treat my grandson the way I should have treated you.' I thought that was great. It also made me feel that *yes*, maybe I could have a relationship with my mother. Maybe it wasn't too late for us to bond.

"Unfortunately, it never happened, maybe because of all the other stuff that was going on, including the way I had dropped out of high school so I could get a job that would provide for my new family. In any case, we lived five minutes away from my family, but there was no communication. They never came over to the apartment where I lived or anything like that. That hurt me. Not to mention, I felt really devastated when my parents got an *ADT* security system and gave the code to my brother, but not to me. That action, on their part, brought all the old feelings back. I was twenty by then, with a good job that had suddenly began to feel like a dead end. That was why I went to see an Air Force recruiter, who agreed to help me study for my GED so I could enlist. I was doing that when my girlfriend and I began to have problems. We were living together with a new baby and I wanted sex all the time. As the breadwinner, I felt entitled to it—that was what we argued about most of the time.

"'If you love me, you'll have sex with me,' I'd tell her.

"'Why can't we just talk?' she would reply. She wanted more from the relationship than just sex, something that was really hard for me to understand."

I asked Dominique how the arguments made him feel and also how they ended.

"We reached one point where I told her if she didn't give me sex, I'd go out and get it somewhere else. She started crying then, and gave me sex that night. But the fact that I had to threaten her with infidelity in order to get it didn't sit well with me. I had always considered myself ugly because I had a good-looking, light-skinned, green-eyed brother who always seemed to get all the attention. Maybe that's why I felt I had to prove a point when my girlfriend didn't give me sex. Lots of older women were looking at me, at that point, and it felt so good. I ran with it.

"I stayed out with other women every night before going home. When my girlfriend asked me where I had been, I lied and told her I was out with the guys. In fact, I was cheating on her. I justified it by telling myself I was still young, with lots of women paying attention to me, while all my girlfriend and I seemed to do was argue and fight. Our problems got worse as I cheated more and more until I became really arrogant. I still felt like I was competing with my brother because I was having sex with some women his age. I also felt like I was competing with my father, who had done the same thing to my mom."

Dominique continued recollecting about that time in his life as he told me how his father called him out on his behavior.

"My father called me in one day to tell me how upset my girlfriend was with me since I was hardly ever home, and he asked me what was going on. In light of the way he had cheated on my mother, I just got angry with him.

"'How can you sit there and tell me I need to be there for my own family when I can't even get into your house? There have been issues between us—big ones—ever since I was a kid.'" "He tried to bring the focus back to me and my current relationship; but I wasn't having any of that. I walked out and slammed the door behind me. Then I went home and gave my girlfriend a sob story.

"'I apologize for the things I've done.' I only said that to smooth things over. I didn't really mean it. I don't like to have to tell you that, but it's true. That's when we got back together and started having sex again."

I asked Dominique how he felt about sex, in light of his past experiences as an abuser and a victim of sexual abuse.

"I guess I felt that the fewer boundaries there were when it came to sex, the better. Having lived in Europe, where sexuality and nudity are much more acceptable than they are here in the United States, I felt that was the way I wanted to live—no boundaries; anything goes."

Dominique went back to talking about the sex he had with his sister.

"The point is this: I knew it was wrong, but my mother didn't believe me, and my father didn't seem to want to do anything about it, so I started to believe, at some point, that it was okay with him. I was still angry about my father's relationship with my sister. He was always protecting her. I felt that if I needed protection, no one was there for me. Anger was a big part of it, even though I was sexually attracted to my sister. So much had happened with my family that I felt open, exposed, and angry. I wanted to get them back somehow, that was the reason that even though I knew what I had done to my sister was wrong, in many ways, it still felt good. Although, the biggest part of it was sexual. I wanted it, and I did it."

At that point, I asked Dominique what he thought might have happened if his father had handled the situation differently, and perhaps gotten him into therapy.

"I believe that if he had addressed the situation and gotten me into therapy, it would have been less likely that I would have ended up here. I was sentenced to twenty years for my sexual crimes against my sister and my son—I'll tell you more about that later. I have served ten years so far, and I take full responsibility for all my actions. But I believe in my heart that if my father had gotten me help when he found out what was going on, I might not be here right now."

I told Dominique that before we went on to the subject of his son, I wanted to give him the opportunity to say anything he thought might be helpful for people who might be thinking about molesting another person.

"A few things come to mind. In school, when I joined the football team, my grades went from A's and B's, to C's then D's as I transformed myself into the assault machine my coach wanted us all to be. I also felt that whatever I did, God always had my back. I was big on isolation too, as I've said, always spending lots of time alone in my room—which was painted black, by the way. Darkness. I liked the darkness; and then at some point, I started to really need it too. Black walls, a TV, video games – I was using all those material things to try to make myself happy; but really, when I thought about it, *was I happy?* I don't think I was. I think it was just a need to succeed in escaping from reality for a little while. I had also started drinking, back in Europe, and I smoked weed a few times too. Luckily, neither the liquor, nor the weed ever became a big problem. I just enjoyed it. It was another way I escaped from the real world and got away from all my problems."

Dominique went on to talk about the abuse that occurred to his son.

"What happened between me and my son is hard for me to talk about. I went further with him than I did with my sister. When my mother told me she was going to treat her grandson the way she should had treated me, that felt good. It felt even better when she did it over the next few months. She would tell him how he was her favorite grandson, then take him out and buy him whatever he wanted. Whenever she did that, I couldn't help thinking, *why hadn't she done that for me?* It was then that I began to feel lots of resentment toward my son; a lot of jealousy. Even worse, there was no one I could talk to about the feelings I was having.

"It didn't help that I felt like I was in a dead-end job again. It also felt like my relationship was going nowhere. When I asked myself what would make me feel better, at that point, I had trouble answering the question. Meanwhile, I was working days, while my girlfriend worked nights; leaving me alone to watch my son. I didn't plan it, but one night when I was giving him a bath, I began to do the same things my cousin had done to me. I fondled him when I washed him, then after he got out of the shower and we still had our clothes off, I asked him if he wanted to wrestle. I remember one night, right before I put him to bed, I laid down on top of him; he was on his stomach. He turned around and looked at me like he was afraid. That look made me so mad, I told him not to look at me. I told him that because I wanted to do what I wanted to do. I knew if he didn't stop staring at me, I wouldn't have been able to do it. He looked away, and that night I did the same thing to him I had done to my sister. When we finished, he got up and put his clothes on. No one ever found out what had happened…what I had done.

"Things got worse after that, everything progressed. I got bored with the same routine and I wanted to find new things to do and new ways to justify what I was doing. One of the things I did was blindfold my son, tying his hands behind his back, and taking pictures of him that way; an idea I had gotten from a movie I had watched when I was younger. That movie had portrayed an adult female being raped. My son was just six at the time. After I took some pictures, I tried to penetrate him, but he jumped and I stopped. Then I untied him, removed the blindfold, and helped him put his clothes back on."

I asked Dominique how he rationalized, or tried to rationalize, that behavior.

"The things I did started out with anger and rage. I also had a hidden desire to tell someone they were going to get it, the desire to possess them, to say, 'You're mine.' At some point, I realized that came from my relationship with my mother. My mother and I had all kinds of problems when I was growing up. One example was when I was sixteen and a senior in high school. She told me I had to go get my picture taken, but I wanted to see my girlfriend whom I knew was already pregnant. When my mother wouldn't let it go, or even let me out of the house, I pushed her and she fell. One part of me felt sorry for pushing my own mother down, but another part wanted to say, 'Hey, that's what you get!'

"That kind of anger with my mother wasn't new for me either. I think it began in Europe when she told me and my brother—she promised us really, that she was going to leave my father, but she never followed through. When she did that, I got the message that she was choosing our father over us, and yes, it made me very, very angry."

Dominique went on to talk about how the fact that his father's mistress was also the choir director made everything even worse for him.

"So here we were in church, singing about God loving us, and she was the one directing the choir. She was the one whose face I had to see each time as I sang. She was the same woman who was sleeping with my father. That really bothered me. It felt like such a huge betrayal! That is why I tried to annoy her at practice. I would do little things like not stand up when she told us to stand up, and then sometimes I deliberately sang in the wrong key. I think she suspected I knew what was going on between her and my father, but I don't think she knew for sure. Her son wanted to fight me once for disrespecting his mother. I just looked at him and said, 'You don't even know.' Then I left. Meanwhile, my mother had all these opportunities to leave my father, but she never took one of them. She chose my father over us; especially me. That's the way I saw it."

I asked Dominique if his course of treatment had helped his current relationship with his mother.

"When I first got locked up back in '98, I could see my mother felt guilty about my imprisonment. She came to see me every weekend and it was good at first. We talked, we cried, we laughed. I thought maybe, since so much time had passed, we could have some sort of relationship. We didn't stay close for long. After I came here, she told me she thought my father was cheating on her again. I held her and told her I loved her. I don't know, maybe that bothered her. Whatever the reason, she never came back by herself. Looking back, I believe she might have told my father what she had told me. Maybe that was why she stopped coming to see me by herself."

Dominique went on to talk about his current contact with his family:

"I see my family often; at least some of them. I had a big resentment against my father right around my thirty-third birthday a few months ago. He had been putting the church ahead of me for a while, and then he decided not to visit me for my birthday. He went to take family pictures instead. I saw that as his way of trying to control me, something he had always done, and something I had always resented.

"Every year, my parents would send me a birthday gift in the amount of my age, so that year, the check was for $33. Enough is enough, that's what I told myself before I sent the check back. My parents didn't like that. They took it personally and told me I had disrespected them by sending the check back. A few weeks later, when my father and brother came up to see me, I knew I wanted to talk to my father and tell him how I was grownup, and I didn't want him trying to control me anymore. When I told him that, he turned it all around, blaming me for everything. Then he said lots of things that bothered me. He told me I hadn't changed in the last ten years. Then he said my molestation never happened. He ended up by saying that if I wanted to be part of his family, I had to respect him. I asked him how I could respect him when, according to him, I hadn't changed at all in the last ten years. Then I said I didn't know whether we could have a relationship or not. I know that hurt him, even though he's never been one to show it. Instead of telling me how he felt, he just sat there, and then he told me that he could tell by my body language that I was frustrated.

"That much was true! 'Why can't you just connect with me?' I asked him. Clearly, that was not what he wanted to hear. He got up and walked out. We haven't really had any type of relationship since then, even though I talked to him a few weeks later. I wanted to talk to my mother too, to tell her it wasn't her fault. When she heard my voice and realized it was me on the phone, she hung up. When I called back, my father answered. When I asked him to tell my mother it wasn't her fault, he told me that in order for me to get to her, I would have to go through him. He went on to tell me how he was sure I was telling everyone I didn't have a father, those days. I replied that I never denied he was my father, but I didn't know if I could go back to my family after my release; not when I felt that they were partially to blame for my problems.

"My father reminded me that I needed a place to live. He also told me how my prosecutor had been in contact with him to make recommendations about the length of my prison term. I knew then that he was someone who felt he had to have power over me, even as an adult. That's why I gave him a message to give my mother, and then ended the call.

"I didn't hear from either of my parents until right after Christmas when they sent me a Christmas card with the message: *You're never too old to be told what to do* on the front and: *And that's final* on the inside. I think my father picked it out, but both he and my mother wrote on the card. The message I got was simple: *If you don't do what you're told, you're out in the cold, but God Bless."*

I went on to ask Dominique if he was up to telling me what had happened with his son. He replied that he was.

"I took several pictures of my son in sexual positions, and then I stopped because I was afraid I would get caught. I have often asked myself why I did that to my son. I think it all goes back to anger. The fact was, I had become accustomed to pain from growing up in my family. *If no one cared about me, then why should I care about my son?* That was the reason I took those pictures and saved them, hiding them in a bedroom closet where I didn't think my girlfriend would ever find them.

"One night, I felt like I just couldn't go on – couldn't do it anymore. I moved the pictures to the living room closet where I knew my girlfriend would probably find them. The next day, she went to work without leaving out any food for me. I checked the closet. The photos were gone. I called her job, but I knew she wouldn't be there. I knew she had gone to my parents' house. It turned out that I was right about that. I was also right about the fact that after they saw the photos, my parents knew they had no choice but to call the police. The police came to get me about an hour later, and I told them everything. I confessed to everything."

Dominique was quiet for a few minutes and I broke the silence by saying it sounded like he was ready to try to turn his life around, and I asked how he currently was doing.

"I'm doing great. I feel like I've accomplished a lot here. I've reached Maintenance Level Five, at which point they say you've come to terms with what you've done, and no longer need treatment. I've got a wonderful support team, as well as friends who actually care about me. I hold a couple of positions here in the institution. I can do that because people here don't care about my past, they care about me. I do a lot of opening up to people and sharing…talking about the things that really matter. I've learned a lot about myself, being here. This is also the place where I grew up. I went from a boy to a man. None of it would have happened, unfortunately, if I had never been sent here."

I told Dominique, that it sounded like the only thing he had ever really wanted was to be loved. I also reminded him that people who do bad things are not always necessarily bad people. I promised to relate his story accurately, and told him how, in my book, I wanted him to be the voice of the person who molests, and how I believed his chapter would help my readers gain a deeper understanding of the problem. Finally, I told him it had been an honor and a privilege to speak with him.

Dominique replied, "It's been an honor and a privilege for me too. I had some doubts about doing this when I first heard about it. You know, I've just told you about my experiences here, about how I feel about everything I've done. I'm proud that I've shared my family experiences honestly with you too, instead of reacting and acting out; something I always did in the past."

Chapter Four

Story of a Survivor
By J.L. Whitehead

W hen I received the call from my friend, Sharon R Wells-Simonson, to contribute to her current project, initially I was flattered. It wasn't because I had the opportunity to contribute to a project whose subject matter is held dear to my heart. I viewed this as an opportunity to create a much-needed dialogue around a topic that no one wants to talk about. We dance around the topic of childhood sexual abuse as if it were something that were separate from ourselves. We tend to treat it as something that happens to "other" people...until it happens to us or someone that we know.

Men of color particularly don't like raising this issue because its concept goes against everything that we have been taught as men...regardless if the man is gay or straight. We have been brought up to be leaders and protectors. We are husbands, fathers, uncles, cousins, sons, and nephews, and yet...in none of that do we identify as being a victim.

I still have a problem with that being part of my identity because a man is supposed to be strong. We are supposed to be the rock that keeps our families together. We are to guide our sons and daughters into the journey that they will embark in called "life;" and yet for many of us – we have this dark secret that we will not share with anyone, not even with the ones closest to us.

I was abused at the age of six, and then again at the age of thirteen. When I was thirteen, I was abused by three different pedophiles who used three different grooming methods. As a child, I was susceptible to all of them. One of my abusers used love, laughter, and perceived honesty to gain my trust. The second used his authority over me to get me to submit to his wants. The last used blatant manipulation.

One of the ways that I addressed the trauma that occurred was to admit that it was trauma to begin with. Men and boys don't admit to this because it goes against who we were brought up to be. Instead of addressing what took place, we will bury it within the recesses of our mind and pretend that it never happened. Admittedly, I never acknowledged what took place. I compartmentalized each event, not realizing that each event was linked to the other. It wasn't until I reached my fifties before I understood just what happened and what impact it had on me. Those events shaped who I ultimately became…good and bad.

It wasn't until I reached my fifties that I finally had the courage to acknowledge that my last abuser raped me. It didn't matter if I gave consent or not because at the age of thirteen, you don't have the ability to give consent.

Rape is such a strong word and is often identified with the abuse of women. I assure you, it happens to men and boys. It's just that boys don't talk about it. Even now, it is difficult for me to say that this happened to me. But my not being able to say it doesn't mean that the event didn't occur.

Pedophiles groom for silence. They buy the victim's silence mostly by convincing the child that they were willing to participate in the abusive activity. They will buy their silence with gifts and money, or perhaps they will blackmail them. If the child has a physical response…perhaps an orgasm, the abuser will use that to prove to the child that they were complicit in the act, when in fact, the child's response was normal given the nature of the activity.

They will blame the child and use guilt to buy silence. And for the most part, this works. I know because this happened to me.

But something else happens when a child is abused.

Up until the time of abuse, that child's emotional trajectory, barring any outstanding psychological issues, would have been on a path of normality. Their self-esteem would be in a place of appropriate development. But when molestation occurs, the trajectory of who the child would have been has been altered. Something has changed emotionally for the victim. Something has been thrown out of whack for them without their knowledge or consent. For some, it could be anger; for others, it could be the issue of trust. And for others still, it could be self-esteem.

I know that for me, personally, my self-esteem was compromised. I may have had self-esteem issues prior to the event when I was thirteen, but keep in mind that the first time that I was molested was at the age of six.

For me, what was thrown out of whack was the need to be included and accepted. If I perceived that someone was rejecting me in any way, shape, or form, it would feel as if my whole world were ending.

I say this because there are many of us who suffer from affliction. We just don't know it.

I talked to many victims of abuse; admittedly more women than men. I find that for women, the main emotion thrown out of whack is the issue of trust. I've found that for men, the emotion thrown out of whack is anger.

I would imagine that the emotion thrown out of whack for most victims is contingent upon the type of abuse, and the personality of the victim.

I wrote an article about molestation regarding the latest allegations that have been levied against the Catholic Church. I submit it to you because it is well worth the read and it will also provide you with additional information regarding abuse.

The Catholic Church has been rocked by another scandal with charges of a massive cover up of sexual abuse perpetrated by trusted guardians of our children. In the state of Pennsylvania alone there are at least 300 reports of priests abusing children that goes back decades.

I try to understand how this could have happened as this is not the first time that the Church has come under fire for accusations of molestation and a subsequent cover up. And while Pope Francis has condemned the actions made by priests that may be guilty of what they have been accused, he may not know the ramifications of those actions. He may not know how those accusations impact the victims...children that have been scarred for the rest of their lives.

Maybe he should know. Maybe he should sit down with adult survivors that can tell him how they are living life now; how they have been changed, and in those changes made choices that have impacted them adversely. He may not know that life for them may have been filled with challenges and struggles. He may not know that abuse does not end with the initial act; but that it continues, and is echoed in the lives of the survivors; sometimes hiding and resurfacing around corners that may take the member by surprise.

I am an abuse survivor.

And although my abusers were not catholic priests, I can speak to what happens to a survivor on both an emotional and psychological level. I know firsthand what molestation does to a victim and the effects are long lasting.

There is no viable reason why the church would take the position that it should protect the priests as opposed to their victims. In order to understand what is going on, you would have to understand the role that the church played in the lives of their parishioners.

As a boy who was raised in the Catholic Church, I remember the hierarchy of the church very clearly. The '70s were a completely different time. Back then, you had complete and total trust in the pastor of your church. The role of the pastor was not one where he was considered a leader, but it was also one where he was revered. I remember that John Cardinal Krol was the leader of the Roman Catholic Archdiocese of Philadelphia. Although I never met him personally, I was well aware of who he was. I knew that his ranking was well above my pastor. And then there were the nuns...nuns that occupied the role of the principal and teachers within my elementary school. What was clear back then is that you did not question any directive that a nun gave you. If a priest told you to do something, you did it...no questions asked. The clergy was held in high regard. And at that time, I had this unrealistic expectation that they could do no wrong. I was shocked to see a priest have a beer or smoke a cigarette. I was certain that they had a direct road map to God and that they were in some regards better than the average person; that they were incapable of sinning since the rest of us were regarded as sinners that constantly needed redemption. We all assumed that they were leading by example and therefore worthy of the respect and honor that they were given.

A stunning example of the humanness of the deity could be reflected in the Netflix documentary entitled, "The Keepers" in which a nun was murdered to keep the actions of a rogue priest from coming to light.

While this is an extreme example of some of the corruption that may exist in the Catholic Church, one thing that remains crystal clear is that the role of priests and nuns is lost in the fact that they are human; and it is within that humanness that they prone to make mistakes. They have their feelings, emotions, triumphs, and failures despite the fact that they have taken the oath to serve God.

I am not condemning the Catholic Church. I'm condemning the actions that have been taken to protect anyone that would molest a child just as I would anyone who is not a person of the cloth.

The topic is one that makes us uncomfortable. It is a topic that no one wants to talk about. Parents don't want to address this issue because to do so would mean that they failed to protect their child from harm. This is not what this means. A parent cannot protect their child 24/7.

As stated previously, I know firsthand what happens when this happens to a victim. Regardless of whether the abuse was painful or enjoyable; regardless of whether the child has an orgasm or are left in tears, the results are the same...they are traumatized. And the trauma carries from the time of the abuse to adulthood. I know because I have lived this. I have connected the dots regarding what happens when you are molested, to the decisions that you make on the road to adulthood. I know that the abuse always sits in the back of your mind...whether consciously or not.

We may drink too much; sex too much; drug too much...we may act out in ways that we wouldn't think of had the abuse never occurred. Your priorities may have been altered. Your sense of trust may have been changed. We may be prone to bouts of anger or depression and don't know why.

I know because this happened to me.

The person that I would have been died in that bed fifty years ago. I have no idea who I would have been because that person no longer exists. Instead, I am left with the man that I ultimately became. I know that I have made many mistakes...mistakes that I can't take back. But I have also made good choices throughout my lifetime.

The thing that I have come to understand is that you are not defined by what happens to you. You are not defined by the mistakes or triumphs that you have made in your lifetime. You are defined by the content of your character. Your mistakes and triumphs are part of who you are. You either learn from the mistakes or you don't.

I've come to understand this over the years.

Most people don't understand the ramifications of molestation. They don't understand what the long-term effects are. They don't understand the dangers of emotional suppression.

But we can address this. We can deal with this. We don't have to remain stuck on the proverbial merry-go-round of whatever negative mindset that we believe comprises who we are. We may need to seek counsel with a professional that may help us to address what has happened to us, and take the appropriate steps to begin the healing the process. It may help us to address the emotions that may have been thrown out of whack for us.

There is healing to be had for all of us. Regardless of the offender, there is light at the end of the tunnel. That is not to be confused with a happily-ever-after type of ending. There is no such thing. We can only continue to fight to be a better person and remember that we are not the sum of what has happened to us. We can only deal with our mistakes and be a better man or woman."

Chapter Five
Sexual Abuse: A Veil of Silence
By Lorraine Elzia

Their lips are sealed in most cases. Shades of chocolate that run the extreme ends of the rainbow of their shared kinship. It's a rainbow of affinity rooted in abuse. For those affected, a heritage rich in strength against all odds teaches them that dirty laundry does not get aired in public; especially in any manner that will bring shame upon the family or against its people in general. So they suffer mentally in silence; under an umbrella of obligation and shame which molds their speech and dictates their actions. The shelter of their silence not only teaches, but demands that they put forth a façade of innocence concerning any violation or first-hand experience of the snatching of their sexual innocent virtue.

Violation is not exclusive to just them, but in the scheme of things, the way "they" deal with it is. Sexual abuse is taboo in general; but speaking of it can be almost sacrilegious in the African American community.

We…don't like to accept that it happens.

We…don't like to acknowledge that it exists.

We…like to think that we are stronger than allowing an infiltration of something so ugly to make its ways into our family boarders or our bloodline.

We…are in denial and subconsciously impart a trait of, "secrecy of the sin" upon our species when it comes to sexual abuse.

A generation of people who have found a way of claiming victory from slavery to a point of soaring to presidential heights has a tough time recognizing, accepting, and dealing with the fact that the crazy drunken uncle that every family has…stepped over the boundaries and laid hands, and other body parts, on the children in the family. Or that *innocent* play between cousins became more than a "kissing cousin" game, and resulted in incestual rape. Or the fact that momma's boyfriend, Aunt Agnus' male friend, or Millie's occasional houseguest, took liberties on the body of a child; but not before threatening that child to keep quiet of what transpired.

Our culture cannot swallow the fact that as we aggressively push forward in all aspects of life to show that we are not only equal, but superior in some aspects, when it comes to our line of thinking and in our actions as a people…our skeletons still have a bit of flesh and blood to them. Those skeletons are alive and kicking, even if we choose to put them in a closet and pretend that they don't exist.

We all have our cross to bear. That statement seems to reign over our logic sometimes.

A cross to bear? Is the loss of a child's innocence the cross that a culture bears as part of a bigger sign of advancement and growth? Is the sad reality of a few casualties of innocence along the way a bitter necessity, and ultimately something to be ignored as we press toward the higher mark?

The problem in our community does not come in the form of taking a stand and trying to rectify a crime as best we can once we are aware of it. In most cases, the African American community will take on that cause as it has done with most others perpetrated against us individually or against our race. We respond, once attacked, with an unrelenting vengeance once the perpetrator is known. So, the problem is not in *what will we do* once confronted with a violation; the problem comes in our sense of comfort in not wanting to know of the violation in the first place.

We are much more content, as a people, to act like we are ignorant that it may be happening, than we are with being forced to take action. We'll act when forced to; our bloodline dictates we are strong in that regard, but we just would rather not have anyone twist our arm to act.

There lies both the problem and the cure.

In order to stop the abuse, our community needs to not only have its arm twisted by the fact that sexual abuse is running rampant; but we need to have our arms broken, and ultimately put in a cast of undeniable pain before we will be prepared to take it seriously. In order to help our children, we need to pull off our, "ignorance is bliss veil" and be more proactive than reactive.

When it comes to reporting sexual abuse, race does matter. African American women are less likely than white women to involve police in cases of child sexual abuse. Their need to remain behind a veil of secrecy is based upon fears about betraying the family by turning abusers into "the system" and a distrust that they have of institutions and authority figures. So often, they just remain silent, being faithful to their "cross to bear" mentality. That silence results in perpetrators remaining free to assault again.

The saying goes, "Once an abuser, always an abuser." The only way to stop that vicious cycle is to bring the abuse to light. The only way to make shades of chocolate victims cry out and bring their abusers to light is for the African American community to raise their veil of "ignorance is bliss" and instill within its children that they do NOT have a "cross to bear" for their race. We need to be more forceful in allowing them the freedom to not see themselves as a representative of their race and its cause. We need to teach them that they, as individuals, are more important than the big picture. We need to stress that although we will fight to right any wrong that we perceive, it is very important for us to have knowledge of the wrongs in order for us to battle them.

The veil of silence is not golden. If we want to put an end to sexual abuse in our community, we must take the time to instill in ALL of our people that they are not martyrs for a bigger picture of cultural advancement, or a casualty in the pursuit of removing racial shame.

Part III
Taking Back Your Power

Chapter Six
Breaking the Cycle of Sexual Abuse
By Stephen L. Braveman

It seems that every time we turn on the television, listen to the radio, or open our web browsers, we are bombarded by stories of yet another priest, teacher, or parent, sexually abusing a child. We are left wondering if sexual abuse of children is on the rise, or perhaps, is it that we simply hear more about it these days due to an increased awareness of the issue, and the overwhelming presence of data fed to us daily.

Regardless of the source, increased awareness of incidences of childhood sexual abuse has given rise to a huge increase in services being offered to assist those who have been wounded. Rape crisis centers are built, books are written, and films are made. At the same time, ways to deal with the perpetrators have also grown at a tremendous rate. We keep passing new laws, building new prisons, and creating new electronic tracking devices; all in an effort to control and contain the guilty. After all, who doesn't want to protect our innocent children and punish evil wrongdoers?

And yet, sexual abuse of children still continues!

Is there another answer? Another way we can really put a dent in, and maybe, just maybe, stop childhood sexual abuse altogether?

This chapter explores basics elements that perpetuate sexual abuse of children. Particular attention is given to the role of early intervention, in our quest, for that ever elusive "ah-huh" moment that will allow us to be just as successful in ending sexual exploitation and abuse, as we are at putting humans into space, cracking the genetic code of our being, and creating the technology to accomplish such tasks.

BECOMING AWARE OF CHILDHOOD SEXUAL ABUSE

To break the cycle of sexual abuse, we must first identify what exactly it is and recognize that it exists. This may be a task harder than one might think. *Why? And haven't we known about this problem for a very long time?* The answers to those questions are "yes" and "no" simultaneously.

Childhood sexual abuse is certainly not a new thing; it's simply a byproduct of modern times. Researchers have documented countless incidences around the world in which humans have been known to molest children dating back to perhaps, the dawn of our species. This human pattern of abuse is clearly spelled out in *The Universality of Incest* (Lloyd DeMause, 1991). It gives examples of everything from "simple incest"—such as childhood marriage to adults—to elaborate rituals of mutilation for the purpose of sexualizing a particular body part, such as the Chinese tradition of "foot binding" with the purpose exaggerating the sexual quality of a woman's foot, especially the large toe, are described in cultures all around the world. At the same time, we find numerous incidences of "innocent" rituals, in which a culture has historically used sexual contact with children for a "noble" cause. *Gilbert Herdt*; Sambia Sexual Culture: Essays from the Field (Worlds of Desire: The Chicago Series on Sexuality, Gender, and Culture, 1999), describes how the *Semen Warriors of New Guinea*, a proud warrior tribe, ritually passed the strong warrior power of the adult males onto the young warrior to-be boys, by way of having the boys swallow the semen of the adult warriors. It was a very special privilege to swallow semen from the biggest, strongest, and bravest of them all.

As we take a close look at our universal past, we find it is sometimes easy, sometimes hard, to define when sexual contact between children and adults constitutes abuse, and when it constitutes appropriate and perhaps "necessary" honored rituals. As our culture keeps evolving, so does our language and what we apply it to. We need to look at current, localized, and American cultural norms, to define what is and isn't considered child sexual abuse today. We are lucky in that we now have a slew of great books, pamphlets, brochures, articles, and films on this topic, and therefore, we do not need to recreate the wheel. In addition to this current text, two such books stand out from the crowd by describing childhood sexual abuse in a manner that adults can relate. Ellen Bass and Laura Davis's groundbreaking book, *The Courage to Heal: A Guide for Women Survivors of Child Sexual Abuse (1988)* set the tone. It was the first substantial book that both identified what sexual abuse looks like, and at the same time, offered a multitude of therapeutic strategies one can take to heal. Mike Lew's groundbreaking book on the sexual victimization of males, *Victims No Longer (1990),* did the same. In addition, Lew's book opened the door to debunking the myth that males cannot be sexually abused, and lead many male victims toward healing. The original version of *Boyhood Shadows*: *I Swore I'd Never Tell*, made by The Monterey Rape Crisis Center and the MAC and *AVA Motion Picture Company (2008),* helps viewers recognize the unique challenges male survivors of childhood sexual abuse face in a palatable, yet highly informative manner.

CHIPPING AWAY AT THE CYCLE

Debunking myths about sexual abuse is now a therapeutic standard when it comes to self-help and professional treatment. It is also essential if we want to end sexual abuse. The more the victims learn about these myths, the less likely they are to be victimized again, and the less likely they are to go on and repeat the pattern.

One myth is that sexual abuse is always violent. Many are surprised to learn that sexual abuse includes non-physical incidences as well, such as being a witness to indecent exposure, receiving obscene phone calls or text messages, being the subject of voyeurism, being exposed to pornography, being a non-physically touched subject of pornography and living in an overly sexualized, emotionally incestual or sexually verbal inappropriate setting *(Laura Davis, 1991)*. In fact, according to the *T.A.S.K. (Take A Stand for Kids)* national website, kissing a child when they do not want to be kissed is considered to be a form of sexual abuse.

The image of what a sexual perpetrator looks like has been changing. Men have, and continue to be, the main culprit in most people's minds. The denial that a female could sexual offend has been very strong. We now recognize that, while at a lesser rate than males, females do commit sexual offenses despite the myth that they are not capable of doing so. Mothers, sisters, aunts, and even grandmothers sometimes molest children *(Scott Abraham, 1997)* and at a rising rate *(Bureau of Justice Statistics, 2002)*. A fairly common occurrence is a female babysitter who explores a young boy's body while changing him and putting him to bed at night *(Mike Lew, 1990)*. Similarly, it is not uncommon for this author to hear female patients report that they were sexually abused by an older female under the guise of initiating the young girl into lesbian love.

Of course, just as with males who molest males, females who molest females are not doing this due to homosexual desire, but rather a desire for power and control over the victim.

Myths about Male Sexual Victimization (Adapted from presentation at the 5th International Conference on Incest and Related Problems, Biel, Switzerland, August 14, 1991), describes dangerous, commonly held myths, specific to males who have been sexually abused as a child. These myths include such things as "the macho image" in which it is believed that boys cannot be sexually abused because they are strong. Of course, boys are children and are not capable of protecting themselves from adults any better than girls. This myth suggests that boys should just tough it out, or "man up," if they are abused. This means he should simply bury the issue and never receive help for it. The myth that only effeminate boys are sexually abused, mixed with the myth that all males who sexually abuse boys are gay, plays havoc on the male victim's sense of self and his sexual orientation. If he grows up to be gay, then his orientation is supposedly caused by the abuse. Both are false in that very "macho" boys get abused at the same rate as not so macho boys. Extensive research has proven that same sex sexual abuse is not capable of causing one to become gay. Another strongly held myth is that boys cannot be sexually abused by females. The false notion that a boy must have an erection to have sex, and that he must want sex to have the erection, falsely leads people to believe that such boy-adult female contact must be consensual. Again, that train of thought is false and damaging in that it allows women to sexually abuse without consequences.

Perhaps the most damaging myth about sexual abuse of children is the one we call the "vampire syndrome," in which, like the victims of *Count Dracula,* once bitten, they will go on to bite others. It is clear to see how this myth is perpetuated. Research has clearly indicated that child victims of domestic violence are very likely to grow up and repeat the pattern if they do not receive help. Research also shows us that approximately sixty percent of career pedophiles were sexually abused themselves as a child. Abuse begets abuse. Logic puts these statistics together to form a perfect storm aimed at the demise of the sexually abused child.

As a result of this myth, many sexual abuse survivors, both male and female, avoid working with children, avoid having children of their own, and sometimes avoid adult relationships all together; all out of unfounded fear that they might abuse the children in their lives. Similarly, many potential partners will call off a wedding or relationship ceremony out of fear that their partner, the survivor, will do such horrendous acts against their own children. However, the truth is far from this logical outcome. In reality, a very tiny percentage of those who have been sexually abused go on to abuse others. Even then, it is common that those who do repeat the crime are mentally ill, developmentally disabled, or still children at the time; meaning that they lack the mental capacity to really know what they are doing. The vast majority of victims/survivors would never abuse a child in this way because logic tells them how bad it was for them, and they vow to never repeat the pattern.

HEALING THE COUPLE:
THE SURVIVOR AND THEIR PARTNER

Just as the alcoholic is likely to relapse if their partner is not involved with treatment, the sexual abuse survivor's odds of acting out, and possibly repeating the pattern of abuse, increase if their partner is not involved in the healing process. Survivors of sexual abuse typically find they cannot establish and maintain a healthy romantic, interpersonal relationship until they've completed significant individual and group psychotherapy. If they've been in a relationship, the relationship has most likely suffered tremendously. Healing for the couple comes through similar means as it did for the individual. Education and confrontation are essential. For example, it's important for both the survivor and the partner to recognize that the partner has now been victimized in the process of being in the relationship, not by the victim, but by the victimization of the victim. Together they have learned how pervasive the damage of sexual abuse can be. Together they can learn how to be partners in the healing.

The handout, *Outgrowing The Pain Together*, by Eliana Gil (1992), is especially useful when read, and discussed in detail, in helping couples coping with sexual abuse healing to understand what they need to do to heal. It addresses the twenty most common issues these couples face. The therapist can help the couple identify which, if any, of these twenty issues the couple still needs to face and it helps develop much of the remaining treatment plan needed based upon the results. As the work progresses, classic and innovative "couple's methods of treatment" may be employed.

EARLY INTERVENTION AND PREVENTION

Two recent projects are breaking the cycle of abuse via early intervention methods. Both of these relatively new programs are showing promising results and may, in fact, be major contributors to ending sexual assaults.

The *Juvenile Sexual Offender Response Team (JSORT)* program, launched in Monterey, California in 2009, offers a new approach utilizing as many public service agencies and departments as possible when a youth is found to have committed a sexual offense. The concept is quite simple: intervene with a youth as soon as it is discovered that he or she has committed a sexual offense. If the child is young and relatively unaware – a "naïve perpetrator" – they are provided with therapy and education. This combination is frequently sufficient to prevent further offenses. If the child is involved with a gang, therapy may occur within the context of group therapy and gang violence reduction programs. If the child is sentenced to time in the Youth Authority, therapy will occur within that setting. While these may sound like commonplace practices, they are actually innovative in that child sexual offenders have typically been dealt with similarly as adult offenders, resulting in punitive measures only—not treatment.

Another highly successful, relatively new kid on the block is the *My Strength Program*. This is a program geared toward keeping non-offending, male teens, from becoming offenders through education and positive group activities. Those who attend this program are given skills to use their own power to say, "No" when their sexual partner asks them "Not to" and to say, "No" when their sexual partner is not in a position to give permission, such as the case when their partner may be intoxicated. Group activities add to the program by providing peer relationships with those who are also taught to be powerful, by saying, "No" to forcing unwanted sexual activity onto a partner.

When combined with other early childhood education programs, such as the *fun music* by Dr. Peter Alsop aimed at very young to puberty-age children, teaching them how to stay "safe" from sexual violence, early intervention programs offer us hope. Perhaps the next generation of children will grow up with a zero tolerance for both being sexually abused, as well as, zero tolerance for becoming sexual offenders.

CONCLUSION

We are realistic. Those of us working in the field of sexual abuse treatment know that we will not see an end to sexual violence and abuse in our lifetimes. We have many who need healing and there is a lot of prevention work that still needs to be done. However, as we teach our children to recognize what sexual abuse is, how to stay safe, how to report sexual abuse if it does occur, and how to be strong and not offend, one day our long-time human pattern of existing with sexual abuse as part of our culture may just perhaps come to an end.

References

Arrien, A. (1991), Lessons From Geese, transcribed from a speech at the Organizational Development Network and based upon the work of Milton Olson.

Bass, E, & Davis, L. (1994), The Courage to Heal: A Guide for Women Survivors of Child Sexual Abuse (third Edition), New York, HarperCollins.

Davis, L. (1991), Healing: When the Person You Love Was Sexually Abused As a Child. New York, HarperCollins.

DeMause, Lloyd (1991), The Universality of Incest, The Journal of Psychohistory, Fall 1991, Vol. 19, No. 2

Gartner. R. B., (1999), Betrayed as Boys: Psychodynamic Treatment of Sexually Abused Men, New York, The Guilford Press.

Gil, E. (1992), Outgrowing The Pain Together, New York, Dell Publishing.

Herdt, Gilbert, Sambia Sexual Culture: Essays from the Field (Worlds of Desire: The Chicago Series on Sexuality, Gender, and Culture), 1999, the University of Chicago Press, Chicago, Illinois.

Hunter, M. (1990), Abused Boys the Neglected Victims of Sexual Abuse, New York: Fawcett, Columbia.

Hunter, M. (1990), The Sexually Abused Male – Vol. 1, Prevalence, Impact and Treatment, New York, Lexington Books.

Hunter, M. (1990), The Sexually Abused Male – Vol. 2, Application of Treatment Strategies, New York, Lexington Books. 5th International Conference on Incest and Related Problems, Biel, Switzerland, (1991)

"Myths about Male Sexual Victimization" (Adapted from presentation),

Geffner, R. (2003), Journal of Child Sexual Abuse, Canada, The Haworth Maltreatment & Trauma Press.

Lew, M. (1990), Victims No Longer, New York, Harper Collins.

Steen, C. (2001), The Adult Relapse Prevention Workbook, Brandon, VT, Safer Society Press.

The Monterey County Rape Crisis Center (2008), Boyhood Shadows: I Swore I'd Never Tell, original release version, the MAC and AVA Motion Picture Company, Monterey, California.

Chapter Seven

The Clean Up After Breaking the Silence
By Lakeisha Shaw Barnes, MA, LPC

As a mental health therapist, I cannot count the number of times that someone has shared a traumatic sexual experience with me followed by the words, "I have never told anyone about this." I then think of all of the guilt, shame, fear, depression, anxiety, and anger – to name only a few emotions, trapped in days, weeks, months, or years of silence. In fact, the more time that passes, the more time those emotions have to extinguish the life out of individuals mentally, emotionally, and spiritually.

It takes a very brave soul to finally break the silence of sexual trauma only to realize that the nightmare of a life that has been lived isn't over. In fact, it is after the silence is broken that the real work begins. We live in a society where everyone is obsessed with DIY projects. In the '80s when a family was trying to replace hideous wallpaper, no one was jumping at the bit to take on that task. *Why you may ask?* Because, despite the desire to get rid of the old, ugly, exterior, what would be found beneath was far worst. Pulling back that wallpaper, piece by piece, exposed a great deal of work to take place before anything new could be established. There is always that group of people that seek to have a new exterior without doing the necessary work beneath the surface.

Unfortunately, taking a short cut in most circumstances doesn't result in a finished product that lasts. Without taking all of the necessary steps beneath the surface, greater imperfections rise to the surface. As a result, when a person finally gets up the nerve to rip the first strip (break their silence) they experience freedom coupled with fear, and relief coupled with regret. Uttering the words that someone violated you or stole your innocence is the start to one of the hardest deconstruction projects that you will undergo, and it is NOT suggested that you attempt to do it yourself.

What does deconstruction look like? Depending on who you ask, you could receive multiple ways to deconstruct and remodel. In my professional opinion, there are some key components to deconstructing in a manner that allows for the greatest chance of a remodel that lasts. A strong support system is a necessity. Additional important elements to facilitate healing and wholeness is putting language to your experience, re-imaging sense of self, forgiveness, silencing negative self-talk, and recognizing triggers.

A strong support system is a priceless key component once a person has broken their silence concerning sexual trauma. Humans are created to be communal beings. We naturally long to be connected to other people. Despite how challenging relationships can be, connection to others is pivotal to live a full, healthy life. While healing from sexual trauma, it is imperative that the people in your support team understand that your mental, emotional, and spiritual state may be unpredictable. As a result, you will need people on your team that have a high tolerance for uncertainty regarding your mood, thoughts, and behaviors. I would never condone anyone not having boundaries regarding other's treatment of them.

When walking with a family member through their battle with cancer, I often found myself getting angry by their actions. One day, I had an epiphany and that was that my empathy toward that individual needed to be much greater than my offense. I loved that person enough to empathize with the pain, fear, and uncertainty surrounding their illness. The people on your team need to be steadfast in their commitment to you and your healing journey.

It is unfortunate that mental health counseling is still a very taboo subject, especially within certain communities, but counseling could be an integral part of finding the long-lasting healing that is often desired after exposing sexual trauma. Finding a professional that you trust to walk you through some difficult memories, cognitions, emotions, and behaviors can be a crucial element of healing. It is important to know that there is a distinction between pastoral counseling and mental health counseling. More often than not, a pastor is not equipped to walk a person through trauma counseling unless they are additionally trained as a mental health professional. Unraveling all of unhealthy coping mechanisms, thoughts, and patterns can take months, and sometime years, to accomplish. Ensure that you establish a dream team of individuals that are willing to walk with you through the messiness of demolition and the rebuilding of your life.

"What's in a name?" Well, to be completely honest, there is a lot of significance in what someone or something is called. Sexual trauma is one experience that I hear people mischaracterize often. In my experience working with individuals that have experienced sexual trauma to call it anything but what it is minimizes the destruction that it leaves behind. Any form of sexual assault or abuse can result in trauma–inclusive of, but not limited to–rape, incest, and molestation. A sexual predator relies very heavily on the silence of the person that has been, or is being abused. It takes courage and strength to reveal the ugly truth of sexual trauma, and even more courage and strength to call it exactly what it is, allowing the maximum potential for re-establishing the innocence and beauty of sexual intimacy.

Whether a person has experienced sexual trauma or not, there is a large number of individuals that have no genuine sense of identity. When a person has been sexually violated and the trauma has been left unhealed, there can be devastating effects on their sense of self. Humans are made of three parts: mind, body, and soul. I teach my clients that a person's identity is also made up of three parts: their public self, private self, and core self. In some cases, there are overlapping characteristics, but depending upon the extent of pain and trauma that a person has experienced, those parts of themselves can be very fragmented.

Our society conditions us to be hyper focused on the part of ourselves that we present to the outside world. Take a moment to ask yourself what characteristics you present to the public. For an individual that has experienced sexual trauma, one or two circumstances usually happen: either a person's brokenness rises to the surface, or a person focuses very heavily on perfecting a mask, not acknowledging, or exposing any imperfections. Both versions are exhausting and usually don't represent who the person truly is.

Private self is self-explanatory. Those are the characteristics that you hold near and dear to yourself or allow only those closest to you to experience. Private self-characteristics may include both positive and negative characteristics. A person who is very in tune with themselves, is honest about their strengths and weaknesses which are most apparent in private settings amongst a small circle of family and/or friends.

Questions usually arise in reference to who we are at our core. I am sure that many can debate me, but I believe that we are all good at our core. I describe to my clients that their core self describes the essence of who they were created to be before being exposed to the world and being shaped by life's experiences. Life experiences, especially trauma related, have the ability to distort or cause dormancy in core characteristics. It is not only important to unearth those characteristics, but to also invest in them in a way that allows them to be most evident publicly and privately. A person must be willing to see themselves as something other than damaged, broken, angry, bitter, resentful, depressed, or anxious. Instead, identify oneself as the beautiful individual that sexual trauma sought to silence and squelch.

Forgive and forget is a statement that quite honestly makes me cringe. *Why?* Because in most cases, unless there is divine intervention or a brain injury of some sort, forgetting is not an option. Forgiveness, however, is. This may be the part of this chapter that makes me unpopular. *Who is it necessary for you to forgive?* My answer is everyone...yourself, your perpetrator, the people who didn't protect you...everyone. *Why is this so important?* Without forgiveness, your life will resemble that of a short-cut deconstruction project.

134

Remember my earlier analogy of the wallpaper? Imagine pulling it all off, but instead of sandpapering away old glue and paper residue, you just place new paper on top. Without forgiveness the residue of your hurt and pain will be evident in how you see yourself and experience others. Forgiveness does NOT mean forgetting, nor does it mean that you are letting anyone off the hook. Well, actually you are. The person that you are letting off of the hook is you – your present, and your future. Forgiveness allows for mental, emotional, spiritual, and physical freedom. You are worth claiming your own freedom from guilt, shame, anger, bitterness, resentment, fear, depression, and anything else that has held you captive due to unforgiveness. Forgiveness is about you; NOT him, her, or them.

One of the most disheartening things to see is for people to not realize that what they say inside their head manifests through their emotions and behaviors. How some individuals think is very heavily influenced by their life experiences. So, imagine all the distortions that are established and reinforced in an individual's thought patterns that has experienced sexual trauma. It is extremely important to stop the record on repeat that says you aren't worthy, aren't good enough, or it was your fault. These are a few common themes expressed by sexual trauma survivors. Living a life of freedom, victory, and wholeness resulting from healing means learning how to recognize, challenge, and change the negative internal dialogue that has plagued your life. Your thought life will require a major overhaul.

The final piece of repair to maintain the mental, emotional, and behavioral beauty of your remodeled self is knowing and understanding the impact of triggers. Triggers are anything or anyone that initiates a negative response in your thoughts, feelings, or body, resulting from your traumatic experience. Recognizing triggers is pivotal in maintaining the healing established after breaking your silence. Once triggers are known, it is important to understand which ones can be eliminated out of your life, and also understand how to minimize your exposure to the ones that can't be eliminated. Once triggered, the use of healthy coping skills and tools will be imperative. Consistent use of healthy coping will help to preserve all of the hard work that has gone into your journey to becoming whole.

The effects of sexual trauma can be devastating. The short or long-term impacts can leave a person feeling empty and broken. Breaking the silence of sexual trauma lessens the damage that secrets are responsible for creating. The good news is that your life doesn't have to remain fragmented. Wholeness is an attainable goal. The unfortunate part is that discovering the new you will require the willingness to let go of the old you. The fact that you have read this book lets me know that you are a survivor because you are still here. Now choose to embark on the greatest remodeling project of your life.

Chapter Eight
Living Beyond the Silence

Denying the reality of abuse does not lessen its effect on the victim or on society. Not all of the affects are as obvious as others, but they are there just the same. Once abused, the victim is never the same. Because of behavioral changes, the effect of child sexual abuse begins affecting the child and the entire family immediately, generally in a negative way. At that point, a rippling affect begins which impacts not only the child, but society as a whole due to actions of the victim.

If they have no love for themselves, what will make them have love for their fellow man?

It makes it easier for a victim to make unwise choices that can be disruptive and destructive to both themselves and those around them. Imagine the impact that it has when measured against more than 42 million adult survivors of child sexual abuse.

One of the most common questions after a victim has broken their silence about being sexually abused is, *what do I do next?* Transitioning from victim to survivor takes much courage, patience, and faith. Although most victims experience similar affects caused by the abuse, the healing journey is one that is unique. Each person heals in a different manner. What works for one victim may not necessarily be the antidote for another. Healing from sexual abuse can be compared to the grieving process. In most cases, as you work through your trauma, you may experience anger, depression, resentment, and hopefully one day, peace, and acceptance. It is not an easy road, but one that is rewarding, and what will free you from the shackles of your painful past. However, as with any illness, you will want to know all of the facts, symptoms, and how it has affected your entire wellbeing. Once you have researched the facts and have identified the areas which have been affected, then you are knowledgeable about what areas to begin working on.

As victims, we have the ability to block out unpleasant and traumatic events in our lives that are too painful to deal with. However, it is not uncommon for the memories of abuse to resurface later in life. The memories have a way of disrupting lives to the point where they can no longer be ignored. Child sexual abuse, unfortunately, has damning emotional and mental effects that many victims carry with them for years or a lifetime. If you are unaware of how the abuse has impacted your life, it's nearly impossible to know where to begin. Seeking professional help soon after the abuse is highly suggested. However, it is never too late to seek professional help so that you can better understand in what areas the abuse has affected you. On the following pages are brief descriptions on the impact of sexual abuse. In addition, I've provided suggestions, questions, and resources that will assist you on your healing journey.

Mental and Emotional Effects of Child Sexual Abuse

Some of the most common effects of child sexual abuse are: guilt, shame, re-victimization, diminished self-esteem, depression, relationship difficulties, and/or other types of dissociative disorders. Post-Traumatic Stress Disorder, (PTSD) is at the top of the list for sexual abuse and childhood trauma. It is a psychiatric disorder that can occur in people who have experienced or witnessed a traumatic event such as a natural disaster, a serious accident, a terrorist act, war/combat, rape or other violent personal assault. People with PTSD have intense, disturbing thoughts and feelings related to their experience that last long after the traumatic event has ended. They may relive the event through flashbacks or nightmares; they may feel sadness, fear or anger; and they may feel detached or estranged from other people. People with PTSD may avoid situations or people that remind them of the traumatic event.

Symptoms of PTSD fall into four categories.
Specific symptoms can vary in severity.

1. Intrusive thoughts such as: repeated involuntary memories, distressing dreams, or flashbacks of the traumatic event. Flashbacks may be so vivid that people feel they are re-living the traumatic experience or seeing it before their eyes.

2. Avoiding reminders of the traumatic event may include avoiding people, places, activities, objects, and situations that bring on distressing memories. People may try to avoid remembering or thinking about the traumatic event. They may resist talking about what happened or how they feel about it.

3. Negative thoughts and feelings may include ongoing and distorted beliefs about oneself or others (e.g., "I am bad," "No one can be trusted"), ongoing fear, horror, anger, guilt or shame, much less interest in activities previously enjoyed, or feeling detached or estranged from others.

4. Arousal and reactive symptoms may include being irritable and having angry outbursts, behaving recklessly or in a self-destructive way, being easily startled, or having problems concentrating or sleeping.

Many people who are exposed to a traumatic event experience symptoms like those described above in the days following the event. For a person to be diagnosed with PTSD however, symptoms last for more than a month, and often persist for months and sometimes years. Many individuals develop symptoms within three months of the trauma, but symptoms may appear later. For people with PTSD, the symptoms cause significant distress or problems functioning. PTSD often occurs with other related conditions such as depression, substance use, memory problems, and other physical and mental health problems (*Diagnostic and Statistical Manual of Mental Disorders, (DSM-5) American Psychiatric Publishing, 2013*).

Depression and Mental Illnesses

Victims who were sexually abused during their childhood are prone to adulthood depression. Research shows that 30-40% of individuals who experienced sexual abuse in childhood report a lifetime history of depression, compared with 10-20% of individuals with no history of child sexual abuse.

Depression is one of the most common mental health conditions in the world. It is more than experiencing trouble getting over a difficulty, or a time of grieving subsequent to losing a friend or family member. It is perpetual sorrow that blocks one's personal satisfaction. Depression frequently includes rest issues, craving changes, and sentiments of blame or lack of concern. Victims may also experience mental illnesses such as personality and dissociative disorders, eating disorders, anxiety, alcoholism, and substance abuse.

Alcoholism/Substance Abuse

Survivors of childhood sexual abuse are at greater risk of developing problems with drugs and alcohol. For some victims, self-medicating is easier than seeking professional help. Because of guilt and shame, victims find it too difficult to ask for help. Self-medicating is sometimes used as a coping mechanism to avoid the painful memories associated with the abuse. Over a period of time, occasional use of substances turn into more frequent use that can eventually lead to addiction. Some may start smoking marijuana to escape everyday reality, others may develop an alcohol dependency, and there are some who may use heroin or painkillers to suppress deep-rooted memories of their abuse. Studies have shown that two thirds of people in treatment for drug addiction have reported being abused as children. According to the American Journal on Addictions, 75% of women who enter treatment programs have reported being victims of sexual abuse. In addition, according to the Journal of Traumatic Stress, an alarming 90% of women who become dependent on alcohol "suffered severe violence at the hands of a parent" or "were sexually abused during childhood." There's no doubt that chemical dependency and alcoholism is often linked sexual abuse. Unfortunately, there is no successful way of suppressing the painful and traumatic horrors of sexual abuse. The only way to move beyond the trauma is by seeking help and assistance to begin the healing process.

Many victims suffer from mental health issues and use drugs and alcohol as a way to cope with mental and emotional issues associated with childhood sexual abuse. The abuse can affect your well-being in these areas:

- Anxiety – Can be associated with fear that the abuse will happen again. It is intense and can cause excessive fear and worry.

- Trust - Abuse may impair your sense that the world is a safe place and impair your ability to trust others. This may be particularly difficult if you had a close relationship with the abuser.

- Self-esteem – You may blame yourself for the abuse, even though it isn't your fault. You may have a hard time feeling good about yourself or hopeful about your future.

- Coping with stress – You may have a lot of negative feelings, which may make it hard to cope with everyday stress.

- Impulsivity – Impulsivity means acting on urges before thinking through the consequences, which can lead to risky activities.

- Anger –You may have a hard time controlling your anger.

- Dissociation – With dissociation, your mind "separates" itself from painful events to protect itself. You may have a hard time remembering what happened, feel like the world around you isn't real, or feel like you aren't connected to your body. It's a common reaction to pain and fear.

- Self-harm – You may harm yourself, but not intend to end your life. It may be a way to cope with difficult thoughts or feelings.

Nurturing Your Inner Child

If you've experienced child sexual abuse, it is very likely that your inner child is wounded. Even when we become adults, we still have the desire to feel loved and accepted. It is not unusual for a child sexual abuse survivor to be angry with their inner child for thinking that they somehow caused or allowed the abuse to happen. They may feel that they could have done something, like tell someone, or have fought back. Some may have tried to quiet their inner voice through drugs, alcohol, self-harm, over-eating, gambling, and other harmful behaviors to avoid confronting the abuse. When the inner child is wounded, the survivor may experience feelings of loneliness, abandonment, anger, and unworthiness.

In order to move forward, it's important to reconnect with that child to understand why we are angry with the child. It's important to learn how to love the inner child before we can begin to love ourselves. This work is extremely important in the healing process. However, it can be painful and hard work, and having a support system or professional before you begin this healing journey is highly suggested.

Reconnecting With Your Inner Child

Before healing your relationship can begin, it is important to acknowledge the feelings that you have about him/her. Accepting and understanding that what happened to you wasn't their fault is very important. Learning to be compassionate, gentle, loving, and kind toward the child is a great starting point. The goal is to bring out your inner child and learn to love it as a parent loves a child. These are some exercises that you can do to help you begin the process:

- Write a letter to your inner child letting them know that what happened was not their fault.

- Reassure them that you will protect them and will keep them safe.

- Sit quietly and embrace your inner child. Let them know you want to learn more about him/her.

- Tell your child that you love them and that you will never abandon them.

- If you quiet your mind, you will hear his or her voice asking for your help. Listen to what the child is telling you.

- Get to know your child, invite him/her to do things with you.

You have to talk to your child several times a day. Only then can healing take place. Embracing your child tenderly, you reassure him/her that you will never let him/her down again or leave him/her unattended. The little child has been left alone for so long.

With practice, you will reconnect with your child in a healthy way, getting to know him/her, and reassuring them that you will never ever leave them.

Journaling

Journaling has great benefits which allows you to get your thoughts and feelings down on paper. It is a powerful way to reconnect with your inner child and to examine your feelings, thoughts, and emotions about your inner child. Writing can help you to understand when and why you've disconnected with him/her. It also gives you the opportunity to release what you are feeling at the present time. Journaling is recommended for individuals who suffer with PTSD, and those who have a history of trauma. It works to improve mental health by helping you to confront challenging events. It helps to become more conscious of what you're feeling (even if you cannot name the feeling). It will also help to move you from a negative mindset to a more positive one. Here are some suggestions that can guide you while journaling:

Find a quiet place away from all distractions.

- Write as often as possible to keep a log of your feelings and your thoughts.

- After you've journaled, reflect on what you've written and let it sink in.

- If you're writing to uncover any sort of trauma, take your time, and go easy. It's not necessary to purge all the details all at one.

- Choose a style of journaling that is comfortable for you.

- This journal is for you, and is not necessary for anyone else to read it. Keep it somewhere safe, write freely, and uncover the details at your own pace.

Therapy

There are many benefits to Psychotherapy, it helps individuals cope with a wide range of traumatic experiences. It provides a safe place for you to share; and what is shared remains confidential. Although therapy has its benefits, it takes time and commitment. Building a trusting relationship with a therapist does not happen overnight. The goals of psychological therapy for victims of sexual abuse helps in preventing and reducing PTSD/trauma symptoms, anxiety, depression, and other mental health issues. It also helps the victim to build self-confidence and self-esteem. In addition, counseling can allow survivors to find new identities and help them to gain greater fulfillment in their lives. Therapy can also give survivors of sexual abuse the possibility to examine new coping strategies to manage feelings in more healthy ways. Survivors can also suffer from triggers related to the abuse that cause painful emotions to resurface. A therapist can provide you with techniques that will help you manage those emotions in positive ways. The benefits of therapy include:

- Help you understand the meaning of sexual abuse and how it has affected your life and your family.

- Help you to gain self-confidence, self-worth, and inner strength.

- Provide outside resources, (i.e. support groups).

- Reduce symptoms of depression, anxiety, and PTSD.

- Process suppressed memories through support of a professional.

- Teach you healthy ways of coping and eliminate self-destructive behaviors.

- Improve your quality of life and your relationships with others.

- Restore a healthy state of mind for a better quality of life.

- Learn self-care strategies.

- Help focus less on the past and more on a healthier future.

Overall, talking to a therapist can help you rebuild a new perspective in life. Your future does not have to be defined by your past. If you need help taking back your life after experiencing sexual abuse, seeking therapy is an effective way to begin your healing journey.

Support Groups

A support group will help you to realize that you are not alone in traumatic experiences, self-defeating thoughts, and painful emotions. Support groups are a safe place to find the encouragement and understanding you need to let go of a past that no longer serves you. It allows you to share with other survivors like yourself who are overcoming the effects of sexual abuse. Sharing your story can free you from suppressed memories and can also help others too. Seeing other survivors move beyond the abuse, and learning new and healthier ways of coping can be empowering. It can give you hope to move on with your life and help you understand that the abuse was no fault of your own. These groups can be very helpful in allowing you to connect with others who face the same challenges you may be experiencing. The benefits of participating in a support group may include:

- Feeling less lonely, isolated, or judged.

- Gaining a sense of empowerment and control.

- Improving your coping skills and sense of adjustment.

- Talking openly and honestly about your feelings.

- Reducing distress, depression, anxiety, or fatigue.

- Developing a clearer understanding of what to expect with your situation.

- Getting practical advice or information about treatment options.

- Comparing notes about resources, such as doctors and alternative options.

There are many types of support groups available that focus on issues that relate to the effects of abuse. Here are some ways of finding a group that is right for you:

- Getting referrals and recommendations from your doctor, therapist, or trusted friends.

- Going online and search for professional mental health organizations.

- Searching online for peer support groups (Facebook, Meet Up, etc.).

- Checking with local therapy centers to see what type of group sessions are available.

Forgiveness

One of the most crucial elements of healing is forgiving. It is likely impossible to move forward until you forgive yourself and others. Most victims believe that they must have done something to cause the abuse to happen, I believed that too. The reality of it all is that I was an innocent child, and my abusers were adults who selfishly chose to violate me. I had to acknowledge the choices I made throughout my life in order to cope with my pain. They were absolutely unwise choices; but today, I choose to focus on my progress and how far I've come, and not dwell on my past. Until I came to terms with that, it was impossible to move on. I had to get totally honest with myself and acknowledge how the abuse negatively affected my life. We all deserve to be healthy and happy.

Forgiving my abusers was the most difficult undertaking I experienced during my healing journey. Some victims may feel that they may never be able to forgive the person(s) that inflicted hurt and pain upon them. But, forgiveness allows you to free yourself and cleanse your spirit of all anger and hate. Holding on to painful feelings is more damaging to the victim. I will never forget, but I will no longer allow the abuse to keep me bound. I set myself free from the pain that left me broken for many years.

Today, I can live with myself, and I've prayed for the souls of my abusers. This is something that takes time and does not happen overnight. I thought that I was incapable of forgiving, but it has allowed me to move on with my life. I suggest that when you're ready, that you do not do this on your own. Finding a support system, therapist, or someone you can trust is recommended before you begin this undertaking.

Creating a new story for yourself

When you're sexually abused as a child, undoubtedly you are stripped of the freedom in creating your own life story. Someone else, your abuser, has taken the liberty of writing your story for you. But now that the silence is broken and you have found the courage to live your truth, you can rewrite your story. Sadly, you cannot change the story of your past, but you can add healthy new chapters into your life.

Faith is the very thing that kept me holding on. Although I didn't always have faith, once I realized that I had a God that loved me and wanted me to be happy, it gave me the courage I needed to hold on. To this day, faith gets me through some challenging times. I know if it were not for God's love, I would not be here today. Even if you are not a believer in God, it's important to believe that there's a power greater than you that has brought you to this moment.

Building positive self-esteem

When you've suffered any type of abuse, it breaks your spirit and tears you down. After all, abuse is all about power and control. Your abuser wanted to have control over you, leaving you feeling defeated and worthless. This is where you have to rebuild yourself and believe in yourself. Yes, it is easier said than done, but it's possible. You will need to take baby steps in this process. Undoing the damage that has been done can take a very long time. These are some suggestions in helping you to become a healthier you:

- Forgive yourself for something that was not your fault.

- Let go of any shame and/or guilt.

- Believe that you are worthy and your life has a purpose.

- Be encouraging to yourself and know that you can accomplish anything.

- Spend quality time with yourself.

- Focus on the positive things that are in your life.

- Know that you are a survivor and can overcome any obstacle.

- Recognize the positive things about yourself.

- Speak lovingly to yourself.

- Let go of anything that is negative in your life that's not serving you in a positive way (this includes people).

- Allow yourself to feel good about who you are.

- Take care of yourself by eating right, exercising, and getting enough rest. You'd be surprised how this makes a difference in how you feel about yourself.

- Face your fears, now that you've broken your silence, you know longer have to hide.

- Remove the mask, you're beautiful as you are.

- Feed your spirit with positive words and affirmations.

I have developed a series of questions that have helped me to uncover the details of my trauma. Hopefully, they will give you a starting point while journaling, and will help you to begin your healing process. Please answer the questions as honestly as possible and be mindful about minimizing your experiences. These questions were created to help you to open up and help you to take back your power! No one has to see these answers but you. If you feel this may be too painful to do alone, I encourage you to do this with the support of a professional or someone you trust. Please use additional paper to complete your answers if needed.

Questionnaire

- At what age do you recall being sexually abused? Explain.

- Who was your abuser and did you trust him/her? Was it a family member or someone close to the family?

- Did your parent or another adult purposely expose his/her body to you?

- Did anyone have sexual contact with you when you were a child that left you confused or feeling ashamed?

- Were you ever shown sexual pictures or films, or were you ever photographed undressed or provocatively posed?

- How close were you to the person who abused you?

- Please describe specific details of what you remember about the abuse.

- How did you feel after the abuse? Explain (ex: ashamed, afraid, guilty, angry)?

- Have you told anyone about the abuse, if so, did they believe you and support you?

- How long did you endure the abuse?

- Did you block out the memories of the abuse and try to forget that it ever happened?

- How did the abuse affect your behavior and how you interact with others (ex: drugs, prostitution, promiscuity, alcoholism, outbursts of anger, suicide)?

- How would you say the abuse changed your life (ex: trust, intimacy, anger issues)?

- Have you ever sexually abused someone or thought about doing it?

- Do you feel that the abuse has affected your ability to have healthy relationships with others?

- Has the abuse effected your self-esteem and given you a negative opinion about yourself?

- Are you ashamed of your body or being naked in front of others?

- Have you minimized the abuse or tried to convince yourself that it really wasn't that bad?

- Have you ever considered therapy or counseling for the abuse? If not, are you willing to seek the assistance of outside help?

EPILOGUE
By Dr. David Cunha

My testimony would be in terms of the extensive ongoing need to tell these stories so that faint voices of abused victims can be heard and brought into light of healing far far sooner. This will take a radically new and sweeping commitment. Therefore, we all need a willing commitment to re-exam open awareness, plus establishing regular ways of dialogue that consistently always present 'touches that hurt' and 'touches that heal,' 'touches that give' and 'touches that steal.' Plus, a defining moment would that this bravery then begets evidences of actual realizing, and thus a belief that mindset and spirit are predicators of everything in terms of sexuality turning into and processing of progressive addictive patterns of dis-ease and ongoing destructive suffering that eventually spreads itself out; harming persons in ways that exponentially end up affecting numbers collectively that otherwise would not be fathomed.

By underestimating the callous, externalizing, and hyper-sexualizing patterns that build with escalation into sexually addictive processes, combined with and thus failing to take assertive early interventions through turning deaf ears and blind eyes to this problem…we offer little, or no concerted effort society-wide, or faith-based support to the helpless and unsuspecting trusting "little ones."

This work is, however, an attempt and beginning effort, at what hopefully becomes an antidote to stand up to the muting silence, the offended (by the topic), the ones who can't bear the pain of it, and thus need a voice to speak for their own voice, and hurtfully, the ones who would rather be seen as not getting their hands dirty by associating with such a 'controversial' subject.

The American society, and sadly the American church as well, simply put has not been willing to take on this concern with bravery, or in a form that puts the hurt and the victims at the heart of things. Here is a light, a prophetess voice in the wilderness who has no constituents necessarily to buff, but who wishes justly to speak to the real concern of those who are continually being hurt.

As a land of freedom, we must help free silenced victims by meaningfully and convincingly with full support, opening our hearts and minds. This would mean we commit to any and all avenues of understanding and garnering support for them to gain help and safety far sooner and with far more regularity than presently or in the past. The bravery of this book is a beginning that as a single candlelight shared, can spread illumination to willing scores of new hearts and mindsets that may finally offer a kind of dawning new age of brightness.

BIOGRAPHIES

<u>Biography of Stephen L. Braveman</u>

Founder and Director of the Intimacy, Sexuality & Gender Center of Monterey, Stephen has been providing professional top of the field Sex Therapy, Sexual Abuse Therapy and Gender Identity Therapy to the Central Coast of California for over thirty years! Stephen serves the needs of individuals with sexual dysfunctions, those who have been sexually abused, couples struggling with sexual and intimacy issues, Transgender community, LGBTQ+ communities, and the communities of all other sexual and gender minorities. Stephen works closely with the California Victims of Crime Compensation Program.

Stephen's unique Male Sexual Abuse Survivors Group has been meeting for twenty-five years. Cited in such places such as *Rolling Stone*, *Newsweek* and even the *Oprah show*, it is the focus of "Boyhood Shadows," a documentary based upon his work.

To contact Stephen, or find more information about him, his book, *CPR For Your Sex Life*, co-authored with Dr. Mildred Brown, and his psychotherapy practice, visit the Intimacy, Sexuality & Gender Center of Monterey at: www.isgcmonterey.net.

Stephen L. Braveman, LMFT, DST
Licensed Marriage & Family Therapist
AASECT Certified Diplomate & Supervisor of Sex Therapy

Biography of Lakeisha Shaw Barnes, MA, LPC

Keisha Barnes is a native of Sedalia, North Carolina, and a graduate of Fayetteville State University. She earned her Master's degree in Professional Counseling from Liberty University. She is a Licensed Professional Counselor in the state of North Carolina. Keisha has experience in numerous areas of counseling including mood disorders, anxiety, life transitions, women's issues, spiritual issues, trauma, anger management, and marital and family counseling. Biblical principles are commonly integrated in her therapy. Keisha is currently on staff as an individual and couple's therapist at Restoration Place Counseling.

Keisha is an advocate for healthy living physically, emotionally, mentally and spiritually and is motivated by seeing the lives of people transformed. Thus, she has a genuine call to educate and counsel in a bold effort toward self-discovery and awareness to find hidden treasures in each individual. Keisha is committed to helping people ascertain what might encapsulate their mind and heart from pursuing all that God has for them. She utilizes her gifts in an uncanny approach to holistically counsel, teach and train – first biblically and then practically – to help reach the next dimension of life while tapping into gifts and talents that otherwise would have remained dormant.

Keisha enjoys public speaking and training teenage girls, women, and couples. She enjoys running, boot camp, massages, and lunch dates with family and friends as a regular part of her self-care. She is married to Terence Barnes and is the mother of three amazing daughters. Keisha and her husband established and lead a group of other young married couples called Kingdom Covenant Connection (KCC) Marriage Group where they seek to support, empower, and provide accountability for healthy, God-centered marriages. Keisha has the heart of a worshipper and loves to sing. Her newest venture includes starting to write her first of many books.

Biography of Nan Wise, Ph.D.

Nan Wise is a licensed psychotherapist, cognitive neuroscientist, certified sex therapist, board certified clinical hypnotherapist, and certified relationship specialist with three decades of experience. She has a Ph.D. in cognitive neuroscience from Rutgers-Newark. After her training in clinical social work in 1984, Nan went on to study numerous therapeutic modalities including Yoga, mindfulness mediation, Cognitive Behavior Therapy, Gestalt Therapy, Neurolinguistics Programming (NLP), and Eriksonian Hypnotherapy–all tools which she uses to develop personalized therapeutic approaches in consultation with her clients whom she sees as fellow travelers.

Nan's interest in the study of sex stems from her belief that many problems have a root in some form of shame. Nan's commitment to the scientific study of sex stems from her desire to help fill in the disconcerting gaps in the basic science regarding the neural correlates of sexuality. Understanding the basic wiring of the healthy brain is the first step in understanding what may go wrong in the case of sexual disorders and chronic pain syndromes that affect men and women.

Nan Wise, Ph.D.
Licensed Psychotherapist
Certified Sex Therapist, AASECT
Certified Relationship Specialist, The American Psychotherapy Association
Cognitive Neuroscience Researcher, Psychology, Rutgers-Newark
Fellow, The American Psychotherapy Association
Fellow, The National Board for Clinical Hypnotherapists
Board Certified Diplomate, The American Board of Examiners in Social Work

Biography of J.L. Whitehead

J.L. Whitehead has been writing professionally since 1989; initially beginning his career as a contributing freelance columnist for "PGN, Incorporated" located in Philadelphia, Pennsylvania. After writing for the publication for a year, he published his first chapbook of poetry entitled "Universal Words" while enjoying various speaking engagements and poetry exhibitions.

His works includes being a major contributing writer to a book of poetry and prose for African American men entitled "A Warm December" in 1989. In 2002, he became a contributing writer and editor for an online magazine entitled "Never2Funky."

J.L. has been a journalist for a national web site entitled, "The Examiner" as well as contributing to CNN's iReport. Mr. Whitehead has also founded his own publication company that goes by the name, Four Brothers Publications. He has released his first full-length novel entitled *Bruthas,* and has also written the manuscript for his first play based on the characters of his novel. In 2013, *Bruthas, The Final Chapter* was released as the second installment of this family crime drama. Both publications are currently available at www.fourbrotherspublications.com and Amazon.

As of 2018, he is a contributor to DemWritePress which is a website that addresses current political issues of the Democratic Party. www.demwritepress.com. He also contributes/owns the following blogs:

This blog is comprised of commentary as it relates to sexual abuse for survivors in general and men in particular:
https://www.fourbrotherspublications.com/blog

This blog addresses political issues and valued commentary on social issues as they pertain to local communities:
http://thewritermegaphone.blogspot.com

Awards:

The Princeton Literary Review Silver Standard of Literary Excellence for "Bruthas" published August 2011 by Four Brothers Publications

About the Author
Sharon R. Wells-Simonson

Sharon R. Wells-Simonson is an author, entrepreneur, and advocate for sexual abuse victims. She is a beacon of light, and her story will take you to that secret place in her life where she shares her own personal experiences of battling a history of alcoholism, drug addiction, unhealthy relationships, severe depression, and self-hatred. Using her own personal testimony of survival for illustration, Sharon passionately speaks out about prevention and awareness of child sexual abuse. This author of several articles and essays, has written heartfelt, spiritual, and inspirational messages.

Sharon is the founder and CEO of Angel Wings Publications, LLC, and founder of Angel Wings Bridge Foundation; a non-profit organization she established to support and empower sexual abuse victims. The organization serves as a bridge that links victims to professional resources that promote healing through support, education, and spirituality.

Through her projects and published work, Sharon's goal is to help decrease the alarming number of teenage suicides, teenage pregnancies, drug and alcohol addictions, prostitution, depression, and PTSD that is occurring in our youth population.

Resources for Help

Alcoholics Anonymous World Services, Inc.
475 Riverside Drive at West 120th St. -
11th Floor
New York, NY 10115
Phone: 212.870.3400
https://www.aa.org

Angel Wings Bridge Foundation
P.O. Box 5342
Greensboro, NC 27435
http://www.angelwingsbridge.com

Adult Survivors of Child Abuse (ASCA)
The Morris Center
PO Box 281535
San Francisco, CA 94128
info@ascasupport.org

ChildHelp
USA-National Child Abuse Hotline
Childhelp USA National Headquarters
15757 N. 78th Street
Scottsdale, AZ 85260
Phone: 800.4.A.Child / 800.422.4453
(TDD):800.2.A.Child / 800.222.4153
http://www.childhelpusa.org

Darkness to Light
1064 Gardner Road, Suite 210
Charleston, SC 29407
National Helpline: 866.FOR.LIGHT
http://www.darkness2light.org

Family Watchdog Website
https://www.familywatchdog.us

Intimacy, Sexuality & Gender Center of Monterey
494 Alvarado St, Ste A
Monterey, CA 93940
Phone: 831. 375.7553
www.isgcmonterey.net

Justice for Children
1155 Connecticut Avenue, N.W.
6th Floor
Washington, DC 20036
Phone: 202.462.4688
http://www.jfcadvocacy.org

Narcotics Anonymous World Services
PO Box 9999
Van Nuys, CA 91409
Phone: 818.773.9999
Fax: 818.700.0700
https://www.na.org

National Association of Adult Survivors of Child Abuse (NAASCA)
http://www.naasca.org
Phone: 323.552.6150

National Children's Alliance
516 C Street, NE
Washington, DC 20002
Phone: 800.239.9950
http://www.nationalchildrensalliance.org

National Sexual Violence Resource Center Website
https://www.nsvrc.org

New York State Domestic & Sexual Violence Hotline
Phone: 800.942.6906

Public Health Website
https://www.publichealth.org

Rachel Grant, M.A. Counseling Psychology
Sexual Abuse Recovery Coach
Phone: 415.484.5682
www.rachelgrantcoaching.com

Rape, Abuse & Incest National Network
200 L Street, NW
Suite 406
Washington, DC 20036
Phone: 202.544.3064
800.656.HOPE (800.656.4673)
http://www.rainn.org

Rising Hope Clinical Assistance, LLC
510 Northgate Park Dr.
Winston-Salem, NC 27106
Phone: 888.446.7301
info@rhclinical.com

Stop it Now!
351 Pleasant Street, Suite B-319
Northampton, MA 01060
Phone: 413.587.3500
Fax: 413.587.3505
Helpline: 1.888.PREVENT
http://www.stopitnow.com

The National Child Traumatic Stress Network (NCTSN)
11150 W. Olympic Blvd., Suite 650
Los Angeles, CA 90064
Phone: 310.235.2633
Fax: 310.235.2612
https://www.nctsn.org

The National Child Traumatic Stress Network-Duke University (NCCTS)
1121 West Chapel Hill Street Suite 201
Durham, NC 27701
Phone: 919.682.1552
Fax: 919.613.9898

National Child Traumatic Stress Initiative Program Office
Center for Mental Health Services
Substance Abuse and Mental Health Services Administration
Department of Health and Human Services
5600 Fishers Lane
Parklawn Building, Room 17C-26
Rockville, MD 20857
Phone: 877.726.4727

Survivors of Incest Anonymous (SIA)
P.O. Box 190
Benson, MD 21018-9998
Phone: 410.893.33220
http://www.siawso.org

Tree of Life Counseling
1821 Lendew Street
Greensboro, NC 27408
Phone: 336.288.9190
admin@tlc-counseling.com

Women Organized Against Rape (WOAR)
1617 John F Kennedy Blvd,
Suite 800
Philadelphia, PA 19103
24 Hour Hotline: 215.985.3333
https://www.woar.org

Book References

What is Sexual Abuse? ©Copyright 2015 ASCA. All Rights Reserved. Information taken from THE MORRIS CENTER, Revised 7/99, www.ascasupport.org

Diagnostic and Statistical Manual of Mental Disorders, (DSM-5) American Psychiatric Publishing, 2013

https://www.psychologytoday.com/us/blog/trauma-and-hope/201704/overcoming-sexual-assault-symptoms-recovery

https://www.betterhelp.com/advice/abuse/benefits-of-sexual-abuse-counseling

Recommended Reading

Bass, Ellen, Davis, Laura (2008) - *The Courage to Heal: A Guide for Women Survivors of Child Sexual Abuse, 20th Anniversary Edition* - New York: HarperCollins Publishers

Bozelko, Chandra (2018) - *Sexual Abuse Survivors Deserve Help, Not Punishment*

Davis, Laura (1991) - *The Courage to Heal Workbook: A Guide for Women and Men Survivors of Child Sexual Abuse 1st Edition*, New York: HarperCollins Publishers

Duncan, Karen (2004) – *Healing from the Trauma of Childhood Sexual Abuse: The Journey for Women* – Connecticut: Praeger Publishers

Grant, Rachel (2012) - *Beyond Surviving: The Final Stage in Recovery from Sexual Abuse* – Indiana: iUniverse Publishing

Lannert, Stacey (2011) – *Redemption* – New York: Crown Publishing Group

Mann, Mary Ellen (2015) - *From Pain to Power: Overcoming Sexual Trauma and Reclaiming Your True Identity* – New York: WaterBrook

The Morris Center, (1999) – *Survivor to Thriver Manual and Workbook* – San Francisco, CA

Wells, Sharon R. (2011) *Without Permission   A Spiritual Journey to Healing* – New Jersey: Angel Wings Publications, LLC

Whitehead, Jerome L. (2017) – *Groomed* – New York: Page Publishing

NOTES